Formulary of Wound Management Products

(Ninth Edition)

A Guide for Healthcare Staff

Formulary of Wound Management Products

(Ninth Edition)

A Guide for Healthcare Staff

David A Morgan

Euromed Communications Ltd
Haslemere, Surrey

©David A Morgan, September 2004

ISBN 1 899015 54 X

Published by Euromed Communications Ltd., Haslemere, Surrey, UK

Printed in Croatia by Zrinski.

Contents

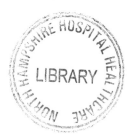

INTRODUCTION

The Formulary of Wound Management Products is a guide to the range of products (mostly dressings) available, their manufacturers and/or distributors, their characteristics and use in wound care. The management of wounds and wound types is also included. Associated/additional information is available in the appendices.

Where possible, evidence-based practice is promoted but there is little evidence to indicate which dressings or topical agents are the most effective in the treatment of chronic wounds. There is good evidence that compression is useful for the treatment of venous leg ulcers. In the treatment of venous ulcers, low adherent dressings are as effective as hydrocolloid dressings beneath compression bandaging. Hydrocolloid dressings are better than wet-to-dry dressings for the treatment of pressure sores[1]. The effects of occlusive and non occlusive dressings compared with simple dressings have not yet been adequately evaluated in randomised controlled trials[2].

A recent Cochrane review on dressings and topical agents for surgical wounds healing by secondary intention identified 13 randomised controlled trials (of small and poor quality). The evidence is therefore insufficient to determine whether the choice of dressing or topical agent affects the healing of surgical wounds healing by secondary intention. Foam is best studied as an alternative for gauze and appears to be preferable as to pain reduction, patient satisfaction and nursing time[3].

Certain treatments, however, appear to be effective but are unlikely to be subject to randomised double-blind controlled trials e.g. dressings promoting moist wound healing. Some of the best treatments available are based on simple observations and are anecdotal. A possible solution in these cases is to develop guidelines in order to support the use of treatments that otherwise would not be prescribed[4].

The Formulary of Wound Management Products will be regularly updated on the Euromed website as new products are launched and further technical information becomes available: http://www.euromed.uk.com/formulary.htm

The information in this booklet is issued on the understanding that it is the best available on the date of compilation. Whilst every effort has been made to ensure the accuracy of the text, no responsibility can be accepted for inaccuracies, omissions or errors. The opinions expressed are entirely those of the author who is a Consultant in Pharmaceutical Public Health, National Public Health Service, Preswylfa, Hendy Road, Mold, Flintshire CH7 1PZ.

KEY:	3M	=	3M Health Care Ltd
	BNF	=	British National Formulary
	DT	=	Drug Tariff
	J & J	=	Johnson and Johnson
	P	=	Pharmacy Only
	POM	=	Prescription Only Medicine
	S & N	=	Smith and Nephew
	TM	=	Trademark in the UK

If the product or a form of the product is available in the Drug Tariff, the symbols (DT) appear after the manufacturer/distributor in the title. For further information see Drug Tariff.

Addresses and telephone numbers of manufacturers/distributors can be found before the index in the BNF. Additional information on Wound Management Products and Elastic Hosiery is available in the current edition of the British National Formulary (Appendix 8)[5].

FORMULARY OF WOUND MANAGEMENT PRODUCTS (A-Z)

3M FOAM DRESSING (3M, DT)
see FOAM DRESSINGS
- a polyurethane foam film dressing with and without adhesive borders
- used for moderate to heavily exuding partial and full thickness dermal wounds
- blue grid and logos show top of dressing to assure pad application to wound
- available in a variety of sizes and styles including a roll for larger wounds; the 8.9 × 8.9cm dressing is fenestrated for tracheotomy tubes and percutaneous tubes or drains

ABSORBENT DRESSINGS
conventional dry dressings e.g.
- **Absorbent Cotton BP:** hospital quality absorbent cotton balls and rolls; should not be used for wound cleansing
- **Gamgee:** pad of cotton wool enclosed in cotton gauze; soft and absorbent; allows strike through
- **Gauze:** open-weave cotton swabs and ribbon; gauze packing is uncomfortable to apply and to remove; capillary loops may grow into fabric of the dressing; when in place it can dry out and harden. Gauze was associated with significantly more pain for patients than other dressings (4 trials). Patients treated with gauze were less satisfied compared with those receiving alternative dressings (3 trials). Gauze is inexpensive but its use is associated with the use of significantly more nursing time than foam (2 trials)[6]
- **Gauze and Cellulose Wadding:** multi-layered cellulose wadding enclosed in absorbent cotton gauze
- **Lint:** cotton cloth with a raised nap on one side and an unlinted wound surface side; not recommended for wound management
- use only on clean dry wounds or as secondary dressings to provide padding or protection over low-adherent dressings
- should not be used directly on the surface of a moist wound
- specifically designed to remove exudate and debris from the wound – highly absorbent

4

- need to be changed frequently (every 12 hours) and skilled nursing care is required
- fail to meet many of the criteria of an "ideal dressing" i.e. they allow strike through, they shed fibres into the wound, they adhere to the wound base and they dehydrate the wound (*see* appendix)

ACETIC ACID
see ANTISEPTICS
- 2–5% solution applied twice daily as a wet-to-dry dressing
- can cause quite severe stinging
- specifically effective against *Pseudomonas aeruginosa* but little effect on other organisms whose numbers may increase[7, 8]
- effectiveness is short-lived
- the activity of this relatively weak acid may be the result of changing the pH of the wound environment, thus inhibiting the organism's growth, rather than a direct bactericidal effect

ACTIBAN (Activa Health Care, DT)
- short stretch compression bandage available in widths of 8, 10 and 12cm (5m long)
- similar to Actico (Cohesive), Comprilan, Rosidal K, Tensolan K, Varex Short Stretch.

ACTICO (COHESIVE) (Activa Health Care, DT)
- short stretch compression bandage

ACTICOAT (S&N, DT)
see SILVER DRESSINGS
- antimicrobial barrier dressing containing a nanocrystalline coating of silver
- dressing consists of 3 layers: an absorbent inner core of rayon and polyester sandwiched between outer layers of silver coated, low adherent polyethylene net. The layers are ultrasonically welded together
- silver is applied by a vapour deposition process, which results in the formation of microscopic 'nanocrystals' of metallic silver. In this form, silver rapidly kills a broad spectrum of bacteria in as little as 30 minutes
- silver content is about 109mg/100cm^2 providing silver in an ionic state at the wound bed in excess of about 70–100 parts per million
- remains effective for a minimum of 3 days depending upon exudate levels
- used over partial and full thickness wounds that may be at risk from infection e.g. pressure ulcers, venous ulcers, burns, donor sites

- dressing is moistened before application with water and kept moist during use to ensure moist wound healing and to enable the silver to exert its antimicrobial effect (do not use saline which interacts with silver)
- can be cut to shape if necessary
- apply the dressing to the wound so that the darker blue side faces the wound and cover with a secondary dressing
- may cause transient discoloration of the surrounding skin
- Acticoat and Acticoat 7 can be used in conjunction with Intrasite Gel in the treatment of chronic wounds (discoloration of the gel is observed)
- dressing is not compatible with oil-based products such as petrolatum
- 5 sizes are marketed but only 2 sizes are available in the Drug Tariff
- **ACTICOAT 7:** a 5-layered dressing consisting of 3 layers of silver and 2 layers of rayon/polyester. Used for partial and full thickness wounds that are critically colonised with bacteria or at risk from infection. Remains effective for a minimum of 7 days depending upon exudate levels. Available in 2 sizes
- **ACTICOAT ABSORBENT:** an Acticoat dressing combined with calcium alginate. Available as a flat dressing and as a cavity rope (for medium to heavily exuding wounds)

ACTI-FAST (Activa Health Care, DT)
- Elasticated Viscose Stockinette
- (Lightweight Elasticated Viscose Tubular Bandage)
- a lightweight plain-knitted elasticated tubular fabric for dressing retention
- washable for reuse
- different sizes available for small, medium and large limbs

ACTIFORMCOOL (Activa Health Care, DT)
see HYDROGELS
- a range of non-adhesive hydrogel dressings containing approximately 70% water
- two-sided, clear, transparent hydrogel formed around a supporting blue polyethylene matrix without an adhesive border
- on dry-lightly exuding wounds, it is recommended that the film top liner of the dressing is left in place; on lightly-moderately exuding wounds, remove the film top liner and apply a secondary dressing
- dressing should be changed when it becomes cloudy or opaque due to the absorption of exudate but may last for up to 7 days
- can be cut to shape of the wound

ACTISORB SILVER 220 (J & J, DT)
see DEODORISING DRESSINGS (formerly called Actisorb Plus)

- 100% pure activated charcoal cloth impregnated with 220mg silver enclosed within a porous nylon sleeve ("charcoal tea bag")
- used for wet or dry wounds where bacterial contamination, infection or odour is present, e.g. fungating lesions, infected pressure ulcers, heavily exuding leg ulcers
- the charcoal adsorbs small gas and liquid odour molecules which reduces the malodour
- active against a wide range of pathogenic organisms including MRSA
- silver produces structural changes within bacterial cells leading to bacterial death
- apply directly to wound surface. If the wound is producing low amounts of exudate, apply a low-adherent dressing first, then Actisorb Silver 220 and an absorbent dressing (which can be replaced whenever necessary)
- can be left *in situ* for 3–7 days, depending on the level of exudate
- should not be cut in order to shape it to the wound site (the dressing is sealed along all four edges); instead the dressing can be folded, easily packed and rolled to fit all wound needs
- can be used under compression bandages
- contra-indicated in patients sensitive to nylon and in wounds that have a tendency to dry out

ACTIVHEAL (film dressing) (Medlogic Global, DT)
see VAPOUR PERMEABLE FILMS

- a vapour-permeable adhesive film dressing
- use on lightly exuding wounds
- has a moisture vapour transmission rate equal to, or better than, the leading brands
- available in the Drug Tariff in 3 sizes

ACTIVHEAL (foam dressing) (Medlogic Global, DT)
see FOAMS

- a polyurethane foam film dressing with and without an adhesive border
- used for moderate to heavily exuding wounds
- good fluid handling capacity and adhesion enabling reduced dressing changes
- available in the Drug Tariff in 3 sizes

ACTIVHEAL (Medlogic Global)

A range of products are available but not in the Drug Tariff:
- a sterile alginate dressing and rope used for medium to heavily exuding wounds
- a cavity dressing used for medium to heavily exuding wounds
- a hydrocolloid dressing used for light to medium exuding wounds
- an amorphous hydrogel dressing used for lightly exuding wounds
- A range of first-aid dressings are available for sale in community pharmacies:
  - Film dressings – for minor cuts, grazes and burns;
  - Hydrocolloid dressings – for minor cuts and grazes which are weeping or bleeding;
  - Alginate film dressings – to aid the control of bleeding from wounds;
  - Skin closures and films – for deeper cuts;
  - Blister dressing with Tea Tree Oil – to prevent or treat blisters;
  - Family first-aid kits – contain a selection of the above dressings;
  - Burn dressings

ACTIVON TULLE (Advancis Medical, DT)

see HONEY DRESSINGS
- a triple layer of folded non-adherent gauze coated with Manuka Honey
- used on partial and full thickness wounds including leg and pressure ulcers, malodorous wounds, dry wounds, sloughy or necrotic wounds
- cover with a low-absorbent secondary dressing and secure with a dressing retention bandage or film dressing
- change at least daily or when the honey appears diluted by exudate
- may be more comfortable if pre-warmed to room temperature prior to use
- promotes moist wound healing, odour control, low adherence and anti-bacterial protection
- due to the osmotic action known to be associated with high levels of sugar, fluid will be drawn from the wound bed
- although there have been no reports of increased levels of sugar in the bloodstream due to the use of honey in wounds, it is advisable to monitor the blood sugar levels of diabetic patients
- do not use if patient is allergic to bee venom
- some patients experience pain through the use of honey on wounds; if pain continues unabated discontinue use of product and irrigate wound with saline solution
- whilst many claims are being made for the therapeutic benefits of Active Leptospermum Honeys e.g. Manuka and Jelly Bush, these and other

varieties of honey are still awaiting further clinical evaluation to determine the full extent of their therapeutic benefits

ACTI-WRAP (Activa Health Care, DT)
- Polyamide and Cellulose Contour Bandage (Nylon & Viscose Stretch Bandage)
- similar to Easifix, Slinky and Stayform
- length 4m stretched
- cohesive and latex free

ADHESIVES (TISSUE)
see DERMABOND, EPIGLU, LIQUIBAND and INDERMIL
- sterile tissue adhesive products containing cyanoacrylate compounds including bucrylate, enbucrilate and mecrylate
- polymerise in an exothermic reaction on contact with a fluid or basic substance, forming a strong, flexible, waterproof bond; in rare cases, the heat may burn
- used for low tension wounds on scalp, face, trunk and limbs e.g. simple lacerations that otherwise might require the use of fine sutures, staples or skin strips
- (wounds under tension need to have appropriate subcutaneous sutures placed prior to adhesive application)
- produces similar cosmetic results to suturing
- a needleless and painless method of wound repair which does not require follow up visits for suture removal; seals the wound and removes the need for dressings
- applied along the length of the wound either in small spots or in a continuous line – avoid adhesive entering the wound; large wounds are closed in sections
- special care is required to ensure that the wound edges are easily aligned so that no adhesive gets between the wound edges; after application, wound edges are held together for at least 30 seconds
- once in contact with the wound, the residual moisture and the natural acids within the skin promote the polymerisation process of the adhesive, resulting in a mechanical bond
- provides the strength of approximated, healed tissue at 7 days, in just minutes
- in the event of accidental adhesion of the skin or lips the bonded surfaces should be immersed in warm soapy water, the surfaces peeled or rolled apart with the aid of a spatula, and the adhesive removed from the skin with soap and water

- compatible with and will not cause irritation to human tissue – there have been no reports of toxicity or carcinogenicity when used topically
- do not use on hands or over joints as repetitive movement or washing will cause the adhesive to peel off
- do not apply to internal organs, blood vessels, nerve tissue or mucous membranes
- do not apply to infected or chronic wounds
- do not use on flexor or extensor surfaces
- used applicators are disposed to sharps or clinical waste
- Indermil, Liquiband and Dermabond adhesives have been compared in terms of ease of use, minimal pain on application, adequate bonding time and wound closure. All produced satisfactory results in terms of wound closure and ease of use. However, Liquiband produced the most consistent results, scoring higher in most of the categories[9]
- a Cochrane Review has concluded that tissue adhesives are an acceptable alternative to standard wound closure for repairing simple traumatic lacerations. There is no significant difference in cosmetic outcome between tissue adhesives and standard wound closure, or between different tissue adhesives. They offer the benefit of decreased procedure time and less pain, compared to standard wound closure. A small but statistically significant increased rate of dehiscence with tissue adhesives must be considered when choosing the closure method[10]
- it is unclear whether tissue adhesives are more or less effective for closing surgical incisions than stitches or adhesive tape[11]

ADVA-CO (Advancis Medical, DT)
see BANDAGES EXTENSIBLE
- latex free type 3c high compression bandage for the management of venous leg ulcers
- bandage has 2 rectangular pressure indicators
  - use small rectangle for ankle circumference of 18–26cm
  - use large rectangle for ankle circumference of over 26cm
- centre line to assist 50% overlap of the bandage
- thin material to promote greater patient compliance

ADVADRAW (Advancis Medical, DT)
- non-adherent capillary action dressing similar to Vacutex
- consists of a soft viscose and polyester mechanically bonded centre, backed each side with a perforated permeable wound contact layer
- acts as a capillary action absorbent wound dressing with a wicking effect similar to Vacutex

- used for medium to heavily exuding wounds
- avoid using on any arterial bleeds or very vascular wounds e.g. fungating wounds
- dressings can be placed side-by-side to cover large wound areas and layered to optimise absorbency
- the integrated central wicking layer absorbs and distributes exudate away from the wound bed
- initially may need frequent changes but can be left in place for up to 7 days depending on exudate levels; will need changing when the top outer layer becomes saturated to the dressing margins
- can be cut to size

ADVAFLEX (Advancis Medical)
- a non-adhesive fixation system for securing bandages
- micro-hook bandage fixation
- suitable for a wide range of bandages, particularly knitted bandages and those with a fibrous surface; not suitable for tightly woven bandages or those with a coating
- available in boxes of 200 tabs on a reel

ADVASIL (Advancis Medical, DT)
see SILICONE DRESSINGS
- a silicone gel sheet combined with a polyurethane film layer (similar to Cica-Care, Mepiform and Silgel)
- for the prevention and treatment of keloid and hypertrophic scars
- self-securing with a gentle release factor
- not to be used on broken skin or wounds
- blue liner is removed and the gel side placed on the scar
- initially applied for a maximum of 2 hours on the first day, increasing by 2 hours per day until comfortably worn for 24 hours
- can be cut to size
- dressing should be removed and washed at least once a day with warm water and mild soap
- re-useable for up to 28 days (discard when the gel starts to disintegrate)

ADVASOFT (Advancis Medical, DT)
- 40% polyester/60% viscose (cellulose) under padding
- used as sub-compression wadding bandage
- used to re-distribute pressure under compression bandages and/or the protection of bony prominences
- soft and conforming

ADVAZORB (Advancis Medical, DT)
see FOAM DRESSINGS
- a hydrophilic polyurethane foam film dressing without an adhesive border
- used for moderate to heavily exuding wounds
- can be left in place for up to 3 days
- 2 sizes available

AEROSOL SPRAYS
see BETADINE, OPSITE, SPRILON
- these have become popular in the last 25 years because of cheap, disposable aerosol cans
- it is difficult to control the uniformity of spray
- they are unsafe to use on the face – there is a risk of eye damage
- multiple-antibiotic sprays containing agents such as neomycin, polymyxin or bacitracin have no place in the treatment of large wounds

ALCOHOL
- fixes skin cells and delays wound healing
- the use of alcohol-based preparations should be restricted to prophylactic skin disinfection before needle insertions or surgical procedures[12]

ALGINATE DRESSINGS
see ACTIVHEAL, ALGISITE M, ALGOSTERIL, ARGLAES ISLAND, COMFEEL PLUS, CONTREET, CURASORB, KALTOSTAT, MELGISORB, NU-GEL, PURILON, SEASORB SOFT, SORBALGON, SORBSAN, SUPRASORB A, TEGAGEN, TRIONIC, URGOSORB [13, 14, 15]
- manufactured from various varieties of seaweeds which contain large quantities of alginates. Seaweeds have been used for many generations by sailors as dressings for wounds
- alginic acid consists of a polymer containing mannuronic and guluronic acid residues. Alginates rich in mannuronic acid (like Sorbsan, Algisite M, Tegagen) form soft flexible gels which can be rinsed away whereas those which are rich in guluronic acid (like Kaltostat) form firmer gels making removal in one piece, easy
- some dressings contain:
  - calcium alginate e.g. Algisite M, Algosteril, Arglaes Island, Seasorb Soft, Sorbalgon, Sorbsan, Suprasorb, Tegagen,
  - calcium-sodium alginate e.g. Activheal, Curasorb, Kaltostat, Melgisorb
  - alginate-hydrocolloid combinations e.g. Comfeel Plus, SeaSorb Soft, Urgosorb

- alginate-hydrogel combinations e.g. Nu-Gel, Purilon
- characteristics of a good alginate dressing are absorbency and wet strength (can be removed without leaving residues in the wound)
- when in contact with wound secretions containing sodium ions, the insoluble calcium alginate is partially converted to soluble sodium alginate through the process of ion exchange (calcium/sodium) into a hydrophilic gel
- highly absorbent – most appropriate for medium to heavily exuding wounds. Only used on exuding wounds as alginates are not suitable for wounds which are very dry or covered with hard necrotic tissue
- can be used on infected wounds
- some have haemostatic properties, e.g. Algosteril, Kaltostat – minor bleeding can be reduced by contact with an alginate for 10 minutes, removal and replacement with another alginate dressing
- should be cut to size or folded over to avoid maceration of the surrounding skin
- do not tightly pack the wound as the fibres expand and the gel will conform to the shape of the wound
- this gel provides an ideal moist environment and allows pain-free dressing changes; the gel ensures that dressing changes do not disturb fresh granulation tissue
- some patients experience a mild "burning" sensation when the dressing is first applied. This may be prevented by moistening the dressing (after application) with sodium chloride 0.9% solution but this will affect the capacity of the alginate to absorb exudate
- recommended that the dressing be changed daily at first then once every 2–3 days or twice weekly as healing proceeds; infected wounds should be changed at least once daily
- most require a secondary dressing (although some have a semi-permeable backing e.g. Sorbsan Plus)
- absorbency and tensile strength of six alginates were assessed in a laboratory comparison. Sorbsan most readily dispersed in saline while Tegagel showed very little tendency to disperse. Kaltostat was intermediate between Sorbsan and Tegagel. Tegagel and Kaltostat are more likely to be removed from the wound in one piece than Sorbsan. The results indicate very different properties which may help in the selection of the appropriate product for a particular wound[16]
- four alginates showed significant differences in important handling characteristics and did not differ significantly in their effect on epithelialisation using a standardised partial-thickness wound model in the domestic pig. More wound fluid was spread laterally with Sorbsan.

Algosteril adhered more than Comfeel Alginate. Kaltostat left more dressing residues on the wound surface at dressing removal than Comfeel Alginate[17]
- histological analysis has demonstrated that prolonged tissue oedema is characterised by the incorporation of alginate (Kaltostat) fibres surrounded by a giant cell foreign body reaction; these fibres seem to disappear as the wound matures[18]

ALGISITE M (S & N, DT)
see ALGINATES
- calcium alginate, non-woven dressing pad and rope containing fast-gelling, mannuronic acid fibres
- made by a needling process which produces a soft, conformable dressing with less fibre shed and high integrity when wet
- used on full and partial thickness wounds with medium to heavy exudate
- absorbs 10 times its own weight in exudate; has significant wet strength and can be easily removed from the wound in one piece
- can stay in place for up to seven days

ALGOSTERIL (S & N, DT)
see ALGINATES
- a sterile, non-woven, calcium alginate dressing
- designed to treat moderately to heavily exuding, infected wounds
- calcium release activates platelets which result in haemostasis
- showed better healing rates than dextranomer paste in a prospective, randomised, controlled trial of 92 patients with full-thickness pressure ulcers[19]
- available as flat dressings and a rope

ALIONE (Coloplast, DT)
see HYDROCOLLOIDS
- a semi-permeable hydrocolloid dressing with or without an adhesive border similar to CombiDERM and Versiva
- consists of:
  - non-adherent wound contact layer with a hydrocolloid adhesive; the non-adhesive dressing has an additional microporous layer for fragile skin
  - a hydrocapillary pad which rapidly absorbs exudate vertically and distributes it horizontally
  - semi-permeable top film providing a water resistant, bacteria proof, MRSA and HIV impermeable barrier

- used for all medium to highly exuding wounds especially where there is a risk of maceration or where dressing changes need to be reduced

ALLDRESS (Mölnlycke, DT)
see VAPOUR-PERMEABLE FILMS
- a protective, absorbent dressing with an adhesive border and a non-woven middle layer (similar to Mepore Ultra and Opsite Plus)
- highly absorbent wound pad
- intended for use as a secondary dressing (although it can be used as a general dressing for medium to high exudate)
- polyurethane backing film which is showerproof
- available in 3 sizes: 10×10cm, 15×15cm and 15×20cm

ALLEVYN ADHESIVE (S & N, DT)
see ALLEVYN and FOAM DRESSINGS
- sterile, polyurethane foam, film dressing with an adhesive border and a low allergy adhesive
- used for moderate to heavily exuding wounds
- can absorb up to 6 times its own weight in exudate
- indicates when it requires changing, without the need for removal (exudate appears underneath the pink film, gradually migrating towards the edges)
- in a randomised comparison comparing Allevyn Adhesive with Granuflex, data indicate that both dressings are easy and convenient to apply; absorbency and ease of removal were better with Allevyn; wear times were similar[20]
- available as square, rectangular and sacral dressings

ALLEVYN CAVITY WOUND DRESSING (S & N, DT)
see ALLEVYN and FOAM DRESSINGS
- made from a matrix of highly absorbent, polyurethane foam "chips" separated from the wound by low-adherent, perforated film
- designed to overcome the problems associated with dressing deep wounds, e.g. pressure ulcers, leg ulcers, surgical incisions and excisions, pilonidal sinuses
- highly absorbent and is designed to manage medium to heavily exuding wounds
- conforms easily to fill cavity
- requires a secondary dressing, e.g. tape, film etc.
- can remain in place for up to 7 days – dressings should not be re-used
- available in DT in circular and tubular shapes
- Allevyn Cavity Wound dressing and Silastic Foam have been compared[21]

ALLEVYN COMPRESSION (S & N, DT)
see ALLEVYN and FOAM DRESSINGS
- sterile, polyurethane foam, film dressing without an adhesive border (formerly called Cutinova Foam)
- consists of a polyurethane top film and an absorbent foam core
- used for moderately to heavily exuding wounds surrounded by sensitive skin
- designed for maximum absorbency under pressure e.g. under compression bandaging
- indicates when it requires changing with the formation of a whitish blister
- available as square and rectangular dressings

ALLEVYN HYDROCELLULAR (S & N, DT)
see ALLEVYN NON-ADHESIVE

ALLEVYN LITE (S & N, DT)
see ALLEVYN and FOAM DRESSINGS
- a polyurethane foam film dressing with a non-adhesive wound contact layer (formerly called Allevyn LM)
- used for granulating wounds with low to medium exudate
- can stay in place for up to 5 days
- can be used in conjunction with compression therapy
- indicates when it requires changing, without the need for removal (exudate appears underneath the pink film, gradually migrating towards the edges)
- square and rectangular, non-adhesive dressings available

ALLEVYN LITE ISLAND (S & N, DT)
see FOAM DRESSINGS
- a polyurethane foam film dressing with an adhesive border
- used for light to medium exuding wounds which may not be suitable for an all-over adhesive dressing
- square and rectangular adhesive dressings available

ALLEVYN NON-ADHESIVE (S & N, DT)
see ALLEVYN and FOAM DRESSINGS
- formerly called Allevyn Hydrocellular
- a hydrophilic, polyurethane dressing with a trilaminate structure:-
  - a three-dimensional, polyurethane, low-adherent wound interface
  - a central hydrophilic, foam, absorbent layer; the foam absorbs and retains exudate not only by capillary action but also by absorption of fluid into the molecular structure of the foam

- an outer polyurethane film consisting of two thin layers of Opsite film
- mainly used on low – medium exuding granulating wounds, e.g. venous leg ulcers
- can absorb up to 10 times its own weight in exudate
- can be cut to shape for use on awkward areas, e.g. heels
- white, patterned face is applied to the wound (pink surface outwards)
- capable of absorbing and retaining large volumes of fluid (several times its own weight) even under a compression bandage
- fluid will not strike through the outer layer but water vapour is lost
- can normally be left in place for about seven days (depending on the volume of exudate)
- indicates when it requires changing, without the need for removal (exudate appears underneath the pink film, gradually migrating towards the edges)

ALLEVYN PLUS ADHESIVE (S & N, DT)
see ALLEVYN and FOAM DRESSINGS
- sterile, polyurethane foam, film dressing with an adhesive border
- used for moderate to heavily exuding wounds
- can absorb up to 6 times its own weight in exudate
- indicates when it requires changing, without the need for removal (exudate appears underneath the pink film, gradually migrating towards the edges)
- available as square and rectangular dressings

ALLEVYN PLUS CAVITY (S & N, DT)
see ALLEVYN and FOAM DRESSINGS
- polyurethane foam, film dressing which is lightly adherent (formerly called Cutinova Cavity)
- very absorbent, highly conformable and can be cut to fit all shapes and sizes of cavity wounds
- available in 3 sizes

ALLEVYN THIN (adhesive) (S & N, DT)
see ALLEVYN and FOAM DRESSINGS
- sterile, polyurethane foam, film dressing without an adhesive border (formerly called Cutinova Thin)
- consists of a polyurethane top film and an absorbent foam core
- used for light to medium exuding wounds where a high degree of flexibility is required e.g. contoured areas of the body
- indicates when it requires changing with the formation of a whitish blister
- available as square and rectangular dressings

ALLEVYN TRACHEOSTOMY (S & N)
see ALLEVYN and FOAM DRESSINGS
- pre-cut dressing for tracheostomy tubes and wound drains

AMNION
see SKIN SUBSTITUTES
- human extra-embryonic foetal membranes composed of:-
  - an inner, amniotic membrane – the amnion, and
  - an outer membrane – the chorion
- amnion is a true biological dressing which is available cheaply if an obstetric unit is on site
- its preparation is time-consuming, tedious and labour-intensive
- adheres to the wound so it is difficult to remove
- not recommended because of the danger of HIV and Hepatitis infection

ANABACT GEL (CHS, POM)
see ANTIBACTERIALS, METROTOP, METRONIDAZOLE
- metronidazole gel 0.75% containing hydroxybenzoates (parabens) and propylene glycol
- use now extended for the treatment of gravitational and pressure ulcers as well as the deodorisation of fungating, malodorous tumours
- apply to wound twice daily
- can be re-used for single patient use up to 28 days

ANAFLEX (Geistlich Pharma, P)
see ANTISEPTICS
- water-miscible cream containing 10% w/w polynoxylin
- polynoxylin is a condensation product of formaldehyde and urea and may act by the release of formaldehyde
- broad spectrum antimicrobial agent active against Gram-negative and Gram-positive bacteria as well as against fungi
- used to treat minor infected cuts and abrasions
- a burning sensation has been reported when applied to broken skin
- applied once or twice a day
- not listed in the BNF as it is "blacklisted"

ANTIBACTERIALS
see ANABACT, FLAMAZINE, METRONIDAZOLE, METROTOP, URGOTUL SSD

ANTIBIOTICS
see BACTROBAN, CICATRIN, FUCIDIN, GRANEODIN
- characteristics of the ideal topical antibiotic:[22]
  - broad spectrum of activity
  - novel mode of action
  - low incidence of bacterial resistance
  - lack of cross-resistance with other antibiotics
  - low incidence of skin sensitisation
  - lack of skin irritation and toxicity
  - acts in the presence of serous discharge
  - not available in a systemic formulation
  - not chemically related to other antibiotics available in systemic form
  - cost effective
- as a general rule, antibiotics should not be applied topically, but given systemically
- there are two main hazards associated with their use – resistance and sensitivity reactions
- controlled use of topical antibiotics will eliminate some of the problems caused by plasmid transfer and induction of antibiotic resistance by inappropriate use; this will reduce sensitivity reactions which can cause considerable harm and delay healing
- multiple-antibiotic sprays containing agents such as neomycin, polymyxin or bacitracin have no place in the treatment of large wounds. Neomycin can be absorbed in sufficient quantities to produce serious toxic effects
- antibiotics are less toxic to cultured human fibroblasts than antiseptics[23]

ANTISEPTICS
see ACETIC ACID, ANAFLEX, BETADINE, CETRIMIDE, CHLORHEXIDINE, INADINE, MEDI-PREP, MERCUROCHROME, PHENOXYETHANOL, POVIDONE-IODINE, PROFLAVINE, SAVLON, SILVER NITRATE, SUDOCREM, UNISEPT, VIDENE
- the ideal antiseptic[24, 25]:
  - is effective against likely contaminants and pathogens
  - kills a wide range of micro-organisms (broad spectrum)
  - is effective over a wide range of dilutions
  - is fast-acting with prolonged residual activity after a single dose
  - is non-toxic, non-carcinogenic and non-teratogenic to human tissues
  - does not easily cause local or systemic sensitivity reactions
  - acts rapidly

- works efficiently, even in the presence of organic material (pus, blood, soap)
- is incapable of promoting bacterial resistance
- has minimal systemic absorption
- is widely available
- is inexpensive
- has a long shelf life
- traditional antiseptics may have toxic effects on tissues and may delay the healing process[23, 26]
- antiseptics are more toxic to cultured human fibroblasts than antibiotics[23]
- avoid alcoholic solutions
- for topical use, antiseptics used judiciously and sparingly are preferable to antibiotics but irrigation of wounds with antiseptics has very little effect[27, 28]
- some antiseptics may be used for short periods only on a rotational basis to avoid the establishment of any particular micro-organism
- chlorhexidine and povidone-iodine are topical antiseptics of choice[27]
- a randomised controlled trial has shown that skin preparation with alcoholic chlorhexidine is more efficacious that skin preparation with aqueous povidone-iodine in reducing contamination of blood cultures[29]
- a paper in WoundCare outlines some of the key considerations for planning the management of a wound using antiseptics[30]
- a review attempts to provide insight into the controversy that surrounds the use of topical antimicrobials by describing their respective mechanisms of action, reviewing supporting evidence and outlining perceived limitations[31]

API-BAN (Apimed, New Zealand)
see HONEY
- contains active New Zealand Manuka honey
- available in single use applicators (15g) for wounds with small openings or multi-use tubes (85g) for application direct onto dressings
- **API-BINE:** active Manuka honey impregnated dressings which are ideal for drier wounds with no slough or where dressings require frequent changing
- **API-NATE:** active Manuka honey impregnated alginate dressings which are ideal for bleeding or sloughy wounds

APLIGRAF (Organogenesis Inc. USA)
see SKIN SUBSTITUTES
- cultured human skin equivalent consisting of combined dermal and epidermal layers

- a bovine collagen fibroblast – containing matrix integrated with a sheet of stratified human epithelium
- also available as Graftskin or Testskin (Organogenesis Inc., Canton, Massachusetts)
- the fibroblasts in the "dermis" and keratinocytes in the "epidermis" are viable, reproducing cells originating from screened neonatal foreskin
- total manufacturing time is about 17–20 days
- morphologically, biochemically and metabolically similar to human skin
- when used as a skin substitute for the in vitro testing of commercial products, Apligraf demonstrated properties similar to those of human skin
- clinical experience is available in treating wounds caused by the surgical removal of skin cancers or keratoacanthomas and in the treatment of venous ulcers
- currently available in Switzerland and North America

AQUACEL (ConvaTec, DT)
see HYDROCOLLOIDS
- a soft, sterile, non-woven pad and ribbon dressing composed entirely of hydrocolloid fibres (sodium carboxymethylcellulose)
- indicated as a primary dressing for the management of medium to highly exuding wounds. May also be used on clinically infected wounds
- applied directly to the wound overlapping the surrounding skin by at least 1cm
- should be changed when it becomes saturated with exudate or by 7 days
- very absorbent – 50% higher than alginates. Converts to a soft coherent gel sheet which retains its integrity during handling
- requires a secondary dressing
- in a randomised trial comparing Aquacel with Kaltostat, the data suggest that Aquacel may have a significantly longer wear time and reduced frequency of dressing change in patients with exuding leg ulcers[32]

AQUACEL Ag (ConvaTec, DT)
see HYDROCOLLOIDS and SILVER DRESSINGS
- a silver impregnated Aquacel hydrocolloid dressing
- a soft, sterile, non-woven pad or ribbon dressing composed of hydrocolloid fibres (sodium carboxymethylcellulose) containing 1.2% silver
- the ionic silver provides up to 7 days of broad-spectrum antimicrobial effect and gives the dressing its silvery colour
- sodium ions in wound exudate bind to the dressing, causing the release of silver ions from the fibres
- bacteria are locked within the gelled fibres and the ionic silver kills bacteria

- used for medium to heavily exuding acute and chronic wounds
- applied directly to the wound overlapping the surrounding skin by at least 1cm
- should be changed when it becomes saturated with exudate or by 7 days
- requires a secondary dressing
- designed not to cause staining
- available as square, rectangular and ribbon dressings

AQUAFLO (Tyco Healthcare, DT)
see HYDROGELS
- a sterile hydrogel sheet dressing without an adhesive border (similar to Hydrosorb, Geliperm and Novogel)
- consists of 23% polyurethane based hydrophilic hydrogel, 47% water and 30% glycols-humectant (moistening agent)
- used for necrotic wounds, dry to moderate exuding wounds and burns
- sheet is transparent and non-adherent
- excellent absorptive capabilities due to its low percentage of water content and high MVTR (8362g/sqm/24hrs)
- will not dry out and can be used in shallow cavities
- use of a secondary dressing is recommended
- available in translucent gel discs (3 sizes)

AQUAFORM (Unomedical, DT)
see HYDROGELS
- an amorphous, starch-based hydrogel consisting of 3.5% starch-grafted polymer in an aqueous base with 20% propylene glycol as an humectant and preservative
- suitable for use at all stages of wound healing from debridement of necrotic tissue to formation of granulation tissue (no exudate to low exudate)
- not suitable for infected or heavily exuding wounds
- requires a secondary dressing
- should be changed at least every one to three days
- gel tends to dry and disintegrate
- sterile, clear premixed gel available in single use 8g and 15g tubes
- the fluid handling properties of Aquaform and Intrasite Gel have been compared in an *in vitro* study[33]

ARGLAES (Unomedical)
see SILVER and VAPOUR-PERMEABLE FILMS
- a controlled release film dressing containing 10% w/w polymer silver ions

which are released at a constant rate until the film is removed from the wound site (5– 7 days); this exerts a constant antibacterial effect
- darker in colour than standard film dressings due to natural tinting of the film by the silver ingredient
- used for the management of medium to heavily exuding wounds
- **Arglaes Post-Op (formerly Island):** a combined Arglaes film dressing with a calcium alginate pad

ASERBINE (Goldshield)
- a mixture of malic, benzoic and salicylic acids in propylene glycol
- used to deslough and cleanse wounds
- has antibacterial properties
- causes cleavage between dead and living tissue probably due to its low pH (2.4)
- may irritate skin around the ulcer e.g. urticarial rash
- during extensive use, wound and skin may become macerated
- available as a solution (the cream has been discontinued)

ASKINA BIOFILM TRANSPARENT (B Braun, DT)
see HYDROCOLLOIDS
- thin semi-permeable transparent hydrocolloid dressing containing carboxymethylcellulose, polyisobutylene and a polyurethane backing
- used for light to medium exuding wounds
- may be left in place for up to 6–8 days (in the absence of exudate) before changing

ASPIRIN
- in a double-blind randomised trial in 20 patients, enteric-coated aspirin 300mg daily, with standardised compression bandaging, improved the healing rate of chronic venous ulcers[34]
- however, the validity of the findings has been challenged[35, 36]

ATRAUMAN (Hartmann, DT)
see TULLE (NON-MEDICATED) DRESSINGS
- a non-medicated, knitted, polyester, sterile tulle dressing
- impregnated with an ointment containing caprylic, capric, stearic triglycerides; caprylic, capric, isostearic, adipic triglycerides (does not contain vaseline or paraffins)
- used for superficial wounds e.g. cuts, lacerations, abrasions
- requires a secondary dressing
- available in 3 sizes: 5 × 5cm, 7.5 × 10cm and 10 × 20cm

AVANCE (Medlock Medical, DT)
see FOAM DRESSINGS and SILVER
- a sterile, silver impregnated, polyurethane foam film dressing without an adhesive border
- silver acts as a broad spectrum anti-microbial killing the majority of bacteria including MRSA
- used on exuding wounds such as leg ulcers and pressure ulcers; not recommended for dry shallow wounds for extended periods because of the possibility of adherence
- dressing changes can be extended to weekly intervals
- **AVANCE A** dressings have a self-adhesive border to keep the dressing in place in awkward areas

BACTIGRAS (S & N, DT)
see CHLORHEXIDINE and TULLE (MEDICATED)
- sterilised Chlorhexidine Gauze Dressing BP impregnated with white soft paraffin containing 0.5% w/w chlorhexidine acetate
- active against a wide range of Gram-positive/negative organisms
- effective *in vitro* and *in vivo* against MRSA
- acquired resistance has been reported
- can be used on large wounds up to 10% body area
- the dressing tends to adhere
- poor release of the chlorhexidine from the hydrophobic paraffin base has been reported when tested by an *in vitro* zone diffusion technique[37]

BACTROBAN (GlaxoSmithKline, POM)
see ANTIBIOTICS
- two different products are available with different uses – they are not interchangeable:
  - sterile 2% mupirocin ointment (polyethylene glycol base) for primary bacterial skin infections (impetigo)
  - sterile 2% mupirocin calcium cream for secondary infected traumatic lesions
- not related to any other antibiotic in use
- active against those organisms responsible for the majority of skin infections, e.g. *Staphylococcus aureus*, including methicillin-resistant strains (MRSA), other staphylococci and streptococci. It is also active against Gram-negative organisms such as *Escherichia coli* and *Haemophilus influenzae*
- there have been reports of spreading resistance to mupirocin among *Staph. aureus*

- applied up to 3 times daily for short courses only (up to 10 days)
- mupirocin (pseudomonic acid) is available exclusively as a topical antibiotic
- side effects are limited to local reactions (in less than 3% of patients) and results indicate that the polyethylene glycol base is the probable causative factor
- sensitisation to mupirocin has so far not been reported
- may be some stinging, burning or itching on application
- used for bacterial skin infections, e.g. impetigo, folliculitis, furunculosis. Its precise place in wound management remains to be established. Limited evidence suggests that mupirocin may be as effective as the current topical antibacterials used but more controlled, comparative studies are needed. Bactroban is probably useful for topical treatment of secondary infected traumatic lesions such as small lacerations, sutured wounds or abrasions (up to 10cm in length or 100cm square in area), caused by susceptible strains of *Staph. aureus* and *Streptococcus pyogenes*

BANDAGES (EXTENSIBLE)[38,39]

- a range of bandages which have extensible properties varying from very low strength for retention of primary wound contact materials, through to strong compression bandages.
- **TYPE 1** (conforming stretch bandages): conform well to body contours and permit free movement of limbs and joints without applying significant sub-bandage pressure. Designed to hold dressings in place and should not be used to apply compression.
  Examples: Crinx, Easifix, K-Band, Slinky, Stayform
- **TYPE 2** (light support bandages, sometimes called short- or minimal-stretch bandages): used to restrict movement and to provide intermittent sub-bandage pressure e.g. to prevent the formation of oedema and give support in the management of sprains and strains. They are not suitable for applying compression or reducing oedema.
  Examples: Crepe BP, Comprilan, Elastocrepe, K-Lite, Knit-Firm
- **TYPE 3** (compression bandages): generally applied to reduce oedema and facilitate venous return in limbs with varying degrees of venous incompetence. The pressure developed beneath this type of bandage is directly proportional to the number of layers used and to the force with which the bandage is applied, but is inversely proportional to the diameter of the limb and bandage width. Compression bandages can be subdivided into 4 groups according to the levels of sub-bandage pressure that they are required to deliver:
- **TYPE 3A** (light compression bandage): able to achieve and maintain low

levels of sub-bandage pressure, i.e. up to 20 mmHg on an ankle 23cm in circumference when applied with a 50% overwrap. Equivalent to Class 1 Compression Hosiery. Indications are for superficial or early varices and varicoses during pregnancy

Examples: Elset, K-Plus, Ko-Flex, MillPlus

- **TYPE 3B** (moderate compression bandages): able to achieve and maintain low to moderate levels of sub-bandage pressure, i.e. up to 30 mmHg on an ankle 23cm in circumference when applied with a 50% overwrap. Equivalent to Class 2 Compression Hosiery. Indications are for varices of medium severity, ulcer treatment and prevention, mild oedema and varicoses during pregnancy.

Examples: Molastic Light, Venopress

- **TYPE 3C** (high compression bandage): able to achieve and maintain moderate levels of sub-bandage pressure, i.e. up to 40 mmHg on an ankle 23cm in circumference when applied with a 50% overwrap. Equivalent to Class 3 Compression Hosiery. Indications are for gross varices, post thrombotic venous insufficiency, gross oedema and ulcer treatment and prevention.

Examples: Adva-Co, Setopress, Surepress, Tensopress

- **TYPE 3D** (extra high compression bandage): able to achieve and maintain high levels of sub-bandage pressure, i.e. up to 60 mmHg on an ankle 23cm in circumference when applied with a 50% overwrap. They are not often used but are indicated for severe lymphoedema.

Examples: Bilastic Forte, Blue Line Varico, Elastoweb

BARRIER FILMS (skin protectants/sealants)
see CAVILON, CLINISHIELD, COMFEEL SKIN CARE, LBF NO STING, OPSITE SPRAY, SKIN-PREP, SPRILON, SUPERSKIN

- protective polymers dissolved in a fast-drying carrier solvent which ideally should:
  - be non-cytotoxic
  - be pain-free on application to broken skin
  - protect skin from moisture, urine etc.
  - protect from skin stripping e.g. adhesive tape trauma
  - be compatible with clothing
- following application, the solvent quickly evaporates, leaving the polymer on the skin
- all of the newer barriers are considerably more expensive than the traditional barriers such as Conotrane, Sudocrem, Drapolene, Metanium and the traditional zinc ointments

BETADINE (Medlock Medical, P)
see ANTISEPTICS and POVIDONE-IODINE
- • wide range of preparations containing povidone-iodine including:
  - antiseptic aqueous solution (10%) – for pre- and post-operative skin disinfection
  - alcoholic solution (10%) – for pre- and post-operative skin disinfection
  - alcoholic paint solution (10%) – used undiluted to minor wounds and infections (twice a day)
  - water miscible ointment (10%) – for skin disinfection (particularly minor wounds)
  - dry powder spray (2.5%) – for skin disinfection (particularly minor wounds)

BIATAIN (Coloplast, DT)
see FOAMS
- polyurethane foam film dressing with or without an adhesive border
- similar profile to other foam dressings e.g. Flexipore, Lyofoam Extra, Spyrosorb and Transorbent
- the adhesive dressing has a skin-friendly hydrocolloid adhesive and a central absorbent pad with a waterproof semipermeable film backing
- the non-adhesive dressing can be used on fragile skin
- used for light to medium exuding wounds
- can be used under compression bandages
- may be left in place for up to 7 days
- range of shapes available including dressings for sacrum and heels

BIOBAG (Vernon-Carus, UK supplier)
see LARVE and MAGGOTS
- sterile larvae supplied in a gauze bag:
  - Mini 2.5 × 4cm – containing approx. 50 sterile larvae
  - Small 4 × 5cm – containing approx. 100 sterile larvae
  - Medium 5 × 6cm – containing approx. 200 sterile larvae
  - Large 6 × 12cm – containing approx. 300 sterile larvae
- sterile larvae are also available in vials
- proteolytic enzymes produced by the larvae diffuse through the gauze and liquefy the necrotic tissue in the wound. This is then reabsorbed into the BioBag and ingested by the larvae
- BioBags should be used on the day of delivery, but if the application is delayed, the BioBag can be stored at 8-10°C for 24 hours
- applied to the wound only, protecting the intact skin if necessary

- the BioBags are covered with slightly moistened gauze, padding and bandages as required depending on the amount of exudate
- it is important to keep the larvae alive during treatment. The BioBags are not covered with an occlusive dressing as the larvae need a constant oxygen supply to survive; direct pressure or a wet environment may make treatment less effective
- during treatment, there is an increase in the amount of exudate, odour and a change in colour (slightly pink) – this is normal
- left in place for 3-4 days; the discarded dressings and larvae are placed in a yellow clinical waste bag and incinerated
- further applications can be made to the wound if necessary
- larvae that have gone through a sterilisation process cannot turn into flies or lay eggs in the wound

BIOBRANE (CliniMed)
see SKIN SUBSTITUTES
- a biocomposite of an ultra thin, semipermeable silicone membrane mechanically bonded to a flexible knitted nylon fabric. A non-toxic mixture of highly purified peptides derived from porcine dermal collagen is bonded to the elastic membrane
- membrane is highly flexible and conformable with excellent adherent properties and a hydrophilic, biocompatible surface; membrane is vapour-permeable
- membrane is applied fabric (dull) side down, wrinkle free against the wound surface with slight tension (using staples or tape to immobilise it). Biobrane is designed to adhere to a properly prepared wound bed and to remain in place throughout the course of re-epithelialisation without changing the dressing
- used for clean partial thickness burn wounds (scalds and donor sites)
- available as
  - **BIOBRANE:** in 4 different sizes
  - **BIOBRANE GLOVES:** available in three different sizes for treatment of hand burns
  - **BIOBRANE-L:** a less complex nylon fabric; available in three different sizes for wounds where less adhesion is desired e.g. meshed autografts

BIOCLUSIVE (J & J, DT)
see VAPOUR-PERMEABLE FILMS
- consists of a thin polyurethane membrane coated with acrylic adhesive
- can be eased apart if it clings to itself during application

BIOTROL DRAINA S FISTULA (Biotrol, DT)
see WOUND DRAINAGE POUCHES
- a wound drainage pouch similar to ConvaTec Wound Manager and Oakmed Option Wound Manager
- used for wound drainage and fistula management
- suitable for wounds with a low – high volume of exudate
- mini (low exudate), small and large pouches (high exudate) are available

BIPP (Aurum)
- Bismuth Subnitrate and Iodoform Paste BPC 1954
- a smooth, yellow, non-sterile paste containing Bismuth Subnitrate BPC (1 part), Iodoform USNF (2 parts) and liquid paraffin (1 part by weight)
- iodoform exerts a mild disinfectant action and bismuth subnitrate has an astringent action but there is no agreement about its mode of action
- used as a mild disinfectant primarily for packing cavities in ENT surgery
- contra-indicated where there is hypersensitivity to iodoform, iodine or bismuth
- bismuth encephalopathy has been reported; some reports have ascribed the neurological effects to the iodoform component
- available as a paste (30g tubes) and impregnated gauze

BLISTERFILM (Tyco Healthcare, DT)
see VAPOUR-PERMEABLE FILMS
- MVTR of 3000g/sqm/24hrs
- 4 different sizes available

BLISTER TREATMENT (SSL)
- non-medicated hydrocolloid absorbent dressing for the treatment and prevention of blisters
- available in small and medium sizes

BURNZAP (Derma Technology)
- a mousse comprising a mixture of paraffin oils and waxes in a spray can
- first-aid treatment for burn injuries which provides local cooling for at least 10 minutes[40, 41]

CADEXOMER IODINE
see IODOFLEX, IODOSORB

CALCIUM GLUCONATE GEL
- a formulation containing 2.5% w/w calcium gluconate and 3% w/w hydroxyethylcellulose as a gel-forming agent with no preservatives was found to be the most appropriate gel for topical treatment of hydrofluoric acid burns[42]

CARBOFLEX (ConvaTec, DT)
see DEODORISING DRESSINGS
- a sterile non-adhesive dressing consisting of 5 layers:
  - ethylene methyl acrylate film (backing layer)
  - absorbent padding
  - activated charcoal cloth
  - ethylene methyl acrylate film (which delays strike through)
  - absorbent wound contact layer containing Kaltostat and Aquacel
- used for the management of malodorous acute and chronic wounds
- may be used as a primary dressing for shallow wounds or with deeper wounds as a secondary dressing over wound fillers
- may be used on infected malodorous wounds under medical supervision together with appropriate antibiotic therapy and frequent monitoring of the wound
- should not be cut to size
- place the fibrous (non-shiny) surface on wound
- with non-infected wounds, may be left undisturbed for up to three days
- available in three sizes: 10×10cm, 8×15cm (oval) and 15×20cm

CARBONET (S & N)
see DEODORISING DRESSINGS
- multi-layered, low adherent, absorbent, deodorising dressing:
  - low-adherent interface of Tricotex
  - absorbent layer of Melolin fleece
  - layer of activated charcoal cloth
- for discharging infected and malodorous wounds
- is highly conformable and can be cut to size
- apply knitted side of dressing to wound

CARBOPAD V C (Vernon-Carus, DT)
see DEODORISING DRESSINGS
- activated charcoal non-absorbent dressing
- consists of a sterile dressing of:
  - low-adherent layer

- an active layer of 100% activated charcoal cloth
- a vapour-permeable film
- a white cover to distinguish the outer side of the dressing; the dark, smooth side of the dressing is placed on the wound
- combines the advantages of a film dressing and an activated charcoal dressing
- used for the treatment of infected, discharging and malodorous wounds
- initially change dressing frequently (1–3 times a day); after 2–3 weeks dressing changes can be made less frequently
- available in two sizes which should not be cut to size

CAVI-CARE (S & N, DT)
see FOAMS
- a conformable foam cavity dressing (formerly known as Silastic Foam)[43]
- a dual sachet dressing consisting of polymers (polydimethylsiloxanes), platinum catalyst, inhibitor and ethanol (10g sachet); polymers, cross-linkers (copolysiloxanes), inhibitor and ethanol (10g sachet)
- the clear fluid contents of the sachets are mixed vigorously for 5–15 seconds. The mixture turns opaque, foams and increases in volume and should be poured into the wound within 30 seconds of mixing. The dressing will set within 3–5 minutes and should not be touched or removed during this period
- skill is needed to mix and mould the stent or bung. The final volume of the stent is approximately four times the volume of the original mixture
- normally used in open deep wounds or cavities of regular shape without underlying tracts or sinuses[43]. It should not be used in dry wounds, mucous membranes, fistulae or sinuses from which the bung cannot be removed; this may lead to a foreign body reaction
- it has the physical and protective functions of gauze packing and is an excellent alternative to packing wounds with ribbon gauze (dressing conforms to shape of wound or cavity)
- a new stent needs to be made approximately every week to allow for wound contraction
- depending on discharge, the stent must be removed from wound at least every 48 hours for rinsing with clean water, soaking in 0.5% aqueous chlorhexidine solution for at least 10 minutes, and then a final rinse with water to remove the antiseptic[44]
- patient manageable; saves nursing time and repeat visits to the clinic
- avoid contact with eyes and with fabric and clothing (it is not removable)
- Silastic foam and Allevyn Cavity wound dressing have been compared[21]
- available in 20g units (2 × 10g sachets)

CAVILON (3M)
see BARRIER FILMS
- a no-sting, protective, transparent barrier film
- indicated as a protective interface between the skin and bodily wastes, fluids and adhesive dressings and tapes (for damaged skin or those with skin at risk of damage)
- provides pain-free protection on broken skin
- is non-cytotoxic and will not interfere with wound healing. It can provide protection for pressure sores, incontinence dermatitis, stoma sites, venous ulcers, adhesion trauma/skin stripping and for peri-wound areas
- applied sparingly - if the "after-feel" is oily, too much has been applied
- product is dispersed in a skin-friendly, non-stinging solvent which is alcohol-free but dries rapidly
- under normal use, requires re-application only once every 48–72 hours
- does not require removal before re-application
- available as a single use foam applicator (1ml and 3ml), as a pump spray (28ml) for larger areas, and in tubes (92g) and sachets (2g)

CELLONA UNDERCAST PADDING (Vernon Carus, DT)
- a sub-compression wadding bandage used as a component of multi-layer compression bandaging
- undercast protection system – protects skin and bony prominences from pressure produced by compression bandages
- water shedding, self conforming, withstands compression, easy to tear
- available in 4 sizes

CELLOSENE (GTM Converting Ltd., DT)
cellulose wadding

CENTRAL GARD (Unomedical, DT)
see VAPOUR-PERMEABLE FILMS
- for central line catheters
- can be used for up to 7 days

CETRIMIDE
see ANTISEPTICS
- a quaternary ammonium compound
- constituent of many products, mostly in combination with chlorhexidine e.g. Hibicet Hospital Concentrate, Tisept and Travasept 100

- has a wide range of bactericidal activity against Gram-positive and some Gram-negative organisms
- 1% solutions are used for their emulsifying and detergent properties especially in A & E Units for dirty wounds
- cytotoxic to mouse fibroblast cells even at low concentrations[45]
- side effects: skin irritation and occasionally sensitisation; should be used with caution – not for routine cleansing of non-infected wounds

CHLORHEXIDINE (many manufacturers)
see ANTISEPTICS

- effective against a wide range of Gram-positive and Gram-negative organisms and some viruses and fungi but not spores. In a comparative trial against 33 strains of methicillin resistant *Staphylococcus aureus* (MRSA), chlorhexidine achieved full efficacy against only 3 strains of MRSA, whilst povidone-iodine was fully effective against every single strain on trial[46]
- 0.05% solutions recommended for wounds; antimicrobial activity may be reduced because of incompatibility, adsorption or in the presence of organic material
- many preparations available e.g:
  - Gauze dressings – *see* Bactigras
  - Dusting powder – *see* CX Antiseptic Dusting powder
  - Chlorhexidine acetate or gluconate 0.05% solutions e.g. Unisept
  - Solutions in combination with cetrimide (*see* CETRIMIDE)
  - Concentrated solutions e.g. Hibitane 5% concentrate
- do not use alcoholic solutions on wounds
- acquired resistance reported with *Proteus mirabilis* and *Pseudomonas aeruginosa*
- side effects: sensitivity may occur, avoid contact with mucous membranes and meninges. A severe allergic reaction has been reported[47]
- a case of acute anaphylaxis, including a widespread erythematous rash, periorbital oedema, sinus tachycardia and mild angio-oedema has been reported after a dressing containing chlorhexidine acetate BP 0.5% was used to dress a burn on a patient's arm[48]
- there is insufficient data to assess safety and efficacy; further clinical trials are required before the use of chlorhexidine on open wounds is either recommended or condemned[49]

CHLORINATED SOLUTIONS
see DAKIN'S SOLUTION, EUSOL, MILTON[50, 51, 52]

- chlorine-releasing solutions are bactericidal to most Gram-positive/negative

bacteria and to some spores and viruses. Their activity is reduced in the presence of organic material and in alkaline conditions
- all solutions cause a moderate to severe irritant response within 4–5 days
- at concentrations recommended for wound cleansing, sodium hypochlorite produces 100% killing of all cell types[23, 53]. Sodium hypochlorite (0.005%) is bactericidal and non-cytotoxic[23]
- are highly toxic to mouse connective tissue fibroblasts
- reduce basal cell viability under certain conditions
- significantly delay the production of collagen and prolong the acute inflammatory response in wounds healing by secondary intention
- may impair epithelial migration
- cause a complete cessation of blood flow
- have a short shelf life e.g. Eusol
- may bleach clothing and other materials
- some advocate the use of these solutions as desloughing agents for 3–4 days only; others prefer to avoid the possible disadvantages by using alternative products having a better reputation (*see* section on Management of Wounds and Wound Types)
- sodium hypochlorite dressing protocols for surgical wounds should be abandoned[54]

CICA-CARE (S & N, DT)
see SILICONE DRESSINGS
- a sterile, soft, self-adhesive, semi-occlusive silicone gel sheet – a cross-linked, polydimethylsiloxane gel
- for temporary use in the management of both new and existing hypertrophic scars (red, raised scars, not flat, white scars). Improves the appearance of red or raised scars
- also used as a prophylactic treatment on closed wounds to prevent hypertrophic or keloid scarring. It is not used on open wounds
- should be applied for 4 hours per day (first 2 days), then 8 hours per day (next 2 days). After this, wear time should be increased by 2 hours per day until a minimum of 12 hours per day is reached (if possible for 24 hours per day). The build up is necessary to acclimatise the skin to the gel sheet
- can be cut to fit the shape of the scar
- best results are usually achieved within 2–4 months
- sheets can be re-used for up to one month. They should be washed twice daily in a mild non-oily soap solution and rinsed in clean warm water
- possible complications are superficial maceration of the skin, rash and pruritus
- available for sale from community pharmacies

CICATRIN (GSK, POM)
see ANTIBIOTICS
- an amino-acid-antibiotic containing neomycin and bacitracin available as cream and dusting powder
- has broad spectrum of antibacterial activity
- may cause emergence of resistant strains
- absorption of neomycin may cause ototoxicity or nephrotoxicity
- bacitracin or neomycin may cause hypersensitivity reactions
- the incidence of allergic contact dermatitis with neomycin is common ranging from 1.7% to 19%
- cream contains wool fat derivatives
- used for superficial bacterial infection of skin but not recommended for wound care

CLEARSITE (NDM UK)
see HYDROGELS
- a hydrophilic, biocompatible gel polymer covered with a polyurethane film marked with a 1cm grid (not removable)
- the gel is approximately 60% isotonic saline solution with approximately 20% propylene glycol and 20% polyurethane polymer
- indicated for treatment of chronic and acute wounds and for wound prevention and protection
- good absorptive capacity whilst maintaining integrity (leaving no residue in the wound)
- can remain in place for up to seven days, while remaining transparent

CLINISHIELD (CliniMed)
see BARRIER FILMS
- wipe on skin protection to protect vulnerable peristomal skin and to reduce skin trauma
- available on NHS prescription

CLINISORB ODOUR CONTROL DRESSING (Clinimed, DT)
see DEODORISING DRESSINGS
- activated charcoal cloth sandwiched between viscose rayon. Both surfaces are identical, consisting of viscose rayon coated with polyamide
- can be cut to size without loss of performance
- applied as a secondary dressing over a primary dressing and secured using surgical tape
- can be re-applied and used for up to 1 week

COD LIVER OIL AND HONEY TULLE (Malam Labs)
see M and M Tulle
- cotton gauze impregnated with cod liver oil, purified honey and 0.5% w/w hexachlorophane

COLLAGEN
see OASIS, OPRASKIN, PROMOGRAN, SUPRASORB C
- fibre-forming protein of mammalian connective tissue (skin, tendons, bones and cartilage) accounting for approximately 30% of the total body protein in mammals
- major component of the extracellular matrix forming an organised structure bridging the basal cells of the epidermis with the adjacent connective tissue matrix
- at least 10 different types of collagen have been identified
- collagen contributes to all phases of the wound healing process:
  - binds blood clotting factors XII and XIII
  - causes natural wound cleansing
  - attracts granulocytes and fibroblasts
  - reduces wound contraction and enhances deposition of orientated, organised collagen fibres
- used as a haemostat, an absorbable suture material, artificial skin, bone filling material and as wound dressings
- there is a slight risk of antigenicity, although this is usually low

COMBIDERM (ConvaTec, DT)
see HYDROCOLLOIDS
- incorporates the technological achievements of super absorbent technology with modern wound care
- a sterile, absorbent, occlusive wound dressing comprising:
  - a polyurethane film
  - Duoderm Extra Thin hydrocolloid adhesive border
  - a non-adherent, absorbent island padding containing superabsorbent polyacrylate granules, which expand and gel in contact with exudate. This holds exudate away from the skin to reduce maceration
  - a non-adherent wound contact layer
- used for chronic and acute, low to medium exuding wounds
- absorbs fluid and retains it within its structure
- resists bacterial penetration for up to 11 days thus reducing the risk of cross-infection
- can be left in place for up to 7 days

- **COMBIDERM N:** non-adhesive dressing used for chronic and acute, low to medium exuding wounds especially in patients with fragile peri-ulcer skin or with sensitivity to adhesive

COMFEEL (Coloplast, DT)
see HYDROCOLLOIDS

- soft elastic pad consisting of carmellose sodium particles embedded in adhesive mass; smooth outer layer and polyurethane film backing
- modified in 1995 to give an enhanced dressing – *see* Comfeel Plus
- available as sheets and as:
- **COMFEEL PASTE** consists of sodium carboxymethylcellulose (NaCMC) and guar gum in a vaseline base; used in conjunction with Comfeel Plus dressings to fill wounds (33% full with paste) with substantial tissue loss (more than 5mm deep); also indicated for debridement of moderate necrosis
- **COMFEEL POWDER** is composed totally of absorbent ingredients: NaCMC, xanthan gum and guar gum. This has high absorptive capacity and is recommended for use together with Comfeel Plus dressings where there are large amounts of secretions, e.g. high wound exudate

COMFEEL PLUS PRESSURE-RELIEVING DRESSING (Coloplast, DT)
see COMFEEL PLUS, HYDROCOLLOIDS

- circular hydrocolloid dressing (semi-permeable) with an adhesive border
- a combination of a Comfeel Dressing and a foam disc with detachable centre pieces attached with microporous tape
- used for light to medium exuding wounds
- used for local pressure relief for existing pressure ulcers and prophylactically in risk sites where local pressure relief is required
- dressing should be changed when the foam backing is reduced to about 50% of original thickness by the effects of compression
- combines pressure relief with moist wound healing
- available in circular and butterfly shapes (especially suitable for heels and elbows)

COMFEEL PLUS TRANSPARENT DRESSING (Coloplast, DT)
see COMFEEL PLUS ULCER, HYDROCOLLOIDS

- a semi-permeable hydrocolloid dressing without adhesive border (transparent version of Comfeel Plus)
- thin layer of transparent, absorbent carboxymethylcellulose with a polyurethane upper film
- used for superficial wounds with low to medium exudate
- the transparent dressing facilitates inspection of the wound
- available in square, rectangular and sacral dressings

COMFEEL PLUS ULCER DRESSING (Coloplast, DT)
see ALGINATES, HYDROCOLLOIDS
- a calcium alginate/sodium carboxymethylcellulose dressing in an elastic self-adhesive mass. Top layer is made from semi-permeable polyurethane film. A calcium alginate/hydrocolloid dressing
- used for light to heavily exuding wounds
- during use the colour of the sheet dressing changes from beige to white to transparent; the dressing should then be changed
- a grid implant on the polyurethane top film provides an easy method for measurement of the wound area
- Comfeel Ulcer and Granuflex products have been compared[55]
- **COMFEEL PLUS CONTOUR DRESSING:** consisting of an oval hydrocolloid core and a four-wing "butterfly" frame of thick hydrocolloid adhesive surrounding the core; for use over awkward areas (sacrum, elbows, knees) and should provide a longer wearing time
- **COMFEEL PLUS SACRAL DRESSING** also available

COMFEEL SKIN CARE (Coloplast)
see BARRIER FILMS
- two products are available:
  - a protective film used by ostomy patients
  - a barrier cream (lanolin-free)

COMPEED HYDRO CURE (J&J)
see HYDROCOLLOIDS
- skin protector patches of various types
- elastic, flexible and waterproof; should be warmed before use
- used to protect areas from blistering or as a first-aid dressing for cuts, grazes, blisters, corns, heel cracks and callouses
- available over the counter

COMPRESSION BANDAGES (TWO-LAYER)
see BANDAGES EXTENSIBLE and PROGUIDE

COMPRESSION BANDAGES (FOUR-LAYER)
see BANDAGES EXTENSIBLE
- a suitable option for patients with venous ulcers but all patients require a thorough assessment

- the four-layer system can be left in place for up to a week
- inexperienced practitioners are more likely to apply dangerously high levels of pressure with single-layer bandages than with a Charing Cross or Profore multilayer system[56]
- little information is available on the maximum pressure that bandages should apply, but a review of the literature suggests that this could be around 60mmHg[57]
- community-based leg ulcer clinics with trained nurses using four-layer bandaging are more effective than traditional home-based treatment[58]
- compression treatment increases the healing of ulcers compared with no compression. Multi-layered systems are more effective than single-layered systems. High compression is more effective than low compression. No clear differences in the effectiveness of different types of compression systems (multilayer and short stretch bandages and Unna's boot) have been shown[59]
- Effective Health Care Bulletin summarises the results of research on the effectiveness and cost-effectiveness of different forms of compression in the treatment of venous ulceration; on interventions to prevent recurrence; and on methods of diagnosing venous ulceration[60]
- in an evaluation of cost-effectiveness of using Profore and Charing Cross systems compared with 'usual care', both four-layer systems were more cost-effective and achieved better healing rates than usual care. Substantial potential savings were identified if four-layer bandaging was used[61]
- the following four-layer systems are prescribable as a kit (rather than single bandages):
  - K-Four 4 layer system (Parema Medical Ltd)
  - Profore 4 layer system (Smith & Nephew)
  - System 4 4 layer system (SSL International)
  - Ultra Four 4 layer system (Robinson Healthcare Ltd)
- typically, components of a multi-layer bandaging system are applied over a wound contact layer and are:
  - First layer: natural orthopaedic wool layer which is used to absorb exudate and redistribute pressure around the ankle. Applied in a loose spiral (2 layers);
  - Second layer: a crepe bandage which increases absorbency and smoothes the orthopaedic wool layer. Applied in a spiral;
  - Third layer: a light compression bandage;
  - Fourth layer: an elastic, cohesive bandage which maintains the four layers in place

- Charing Cross multi-layer system:[62]
  1. Orthopaedic wool such as Velband (J & J) or Soffban (S & N)
  2. Crepe (10cm)
  3. Elset (Seton, 10cm) – elastic, conformable compression bandage applied at mid-stretch in a figure of eight from toe to knee with a 50% overlap
  4. Coban (3M, 10cm) – lightweight, elastic, cohesive bandage applied at mid-stretch with a 50% overlap
- **Hospi-Four (Millpledge Healthcare, DT)**
  1. Ortho-Band Plus – sub-compression wadding bandage
  2. Hospicrepe – cotton stretch bandage
  3. MillPlus – type 3a compression bandage
  4. AAA–Flex – lightweight, elastic, cohesive bandage
- **K-Four (Parema, DT)**
  1. K-Soft – sub-compression wadding bandage
  2. K-Lite – light support bandage (type 2)
  3. K-Plus – a type 3a light compression bandage
  4. Ko-Flex – cohesive flexible bandage
- **Profore system (S & N, DT). For ankle circumference 18–25cm:**
  1. Soffban – natural orthopaedic wool layer
  2. Soffcrepe – crepe bandage
  3. Litepress – a type 3a light compression bandage
  4. Co-Plus – cohesive flexible bandage
  Note: there are 4 other Profore systems available for ankle circumferences less than 18cm, 25–30cm and greater than 30cm; also Profore Lite for reduced compression for mixed aetiology ulcers
- **System 4 (SSL, DT): For ankle circumference 18–25cm:**
  1. Softexe, wadding bandage
  2. Setocrepe (10cm)
  3. Elset (10cm) – elastic, conformable compression bandage applied at mid-stretch in a figure of eight from toe to knee with a 50% overlap.
  4. Coban (3M, 10cm) – type 3b, lightweight, elastic, cohesive bandage applied at mid-stretch with a 50% overlap
  Note: there are also other System 4 combinations for ankle circumferences less than 18cm, 25–30cm and greater than 30cm
- **Ultra Four non-latex bandages (Robinson Healthcare, DT). For ankle circumference 18–25cm:**
  1. Ultra Soft Wadding bandage – applied in a spiral format from toe to knee with a 50% overlap and no pressure
  2. Ultra Lite, crepe bandage – applied in a spiral format from toe to knee with a 50% overlap

3. Ultra Plus, long stretch bandage – applied in a figure of eight format (4 layers) from toe to knee with a 50% overlap at mid stretch
4. Ultra Fast Cohesive Bandage – applied in a spiral format from toe to knee with a 50% overlap at mid stretch
Note: 100% latex free multi-layer bandage system

COMPRESSION HOSIERY[63, 64, 65]

- for those patients who cannot tolerate four-layer bandaging, an alternative is below-knee graduated compression hosiery (mild compression is better than no compression)
- GPs prescribe hosiery from the Drug Tariff which uses the following British classification:

  Class I, Light support, compression at ankle 14-17mmHg (for varicose veins, mild oedema)

  Class II, Medium support, compression at ankle 18-24mmHg (for severe varicose veins, mild oedema, prevention of ulcer recurrence)

  Class III, Strong support, compression at ankle 25-35mmHg (for severe varicose veins, gross oedema, prevention of ulcer recurrence, chronic venous insufficiency)

- hospitals tend to prescribe hosiery which meets a European classification - the pressure applied by the stockings is greater and they are more difficult to use
- there are several types of compression hosiery:
  - circular knit stockings
  - flat-bed stockings
  - net stockings
  - one-way stretch stockings
- hosiery is available in different styles and comes in made-to-measure or standard sizes. A choice of colour is often available. The foot can be either open (easier to apply) or closed toe:
  - below-knee stockings
  - thigh-length stockings
  - thigh-length hold-ups
  - thigh length with waist attachment
  - tights
  - male 'socks'
- only below knee, thigh length and male 'socks' are available on GP prescription
- adopting a systematic approach to assessment will help to identify the most suitable type and class of stocking required

- knee-length stockings should replace thigh-length stockings, being equally effective, cheaper, more likely to fit correctly and better tolerated by patients in the prevention of venous thromboembolism[66]
- patients should be prescribed 2 stockings per affected limb; stockings should be washed frequently and replaced every 6 months
- accurate measurement is essential to ensure a proper fit
- time should be taken to instruct all patients on the correct method of application and how to care for their hosiery
- patient concordance with compression hosiery is problematic e.g. patient's dexterity needs to be considered
- stockings should be worn during the day and removed at night
- compression hosiery should not be used on limbs with an ankle brachial index of <0.8
- analysis of 16 randomised control trials confirm that graduated compression stockings (GCS) are effective in diminishing the risk of deep vein thrombosis in hospitalised patients. The data also suggests that GCS on a background of another method of prophylaxis is even more effective than GCS on its own[67]

COMPRILAN (BSN Medical, DT)
see BANDAGES EXTENSIBLE
- short stretch compression bandage (similar to Silkolan)
- four sizes available

CONOTRANE (Yamanouchi)
see BARRIER FILMS
- medicated cream containing 22% dimeticone and 0.1% benzalkonium chloride
- not recommended as there are blander, less complex products available

CONTREET (Coloplast, DT)
see FOAMS, HYDROCOLLOIDS and SILVER DRESSINGS
- silver containing foam and hydrocolloid dressings
- clinical studies have shown that the dressings kick-start the wound if healing has been delayed or stopped
- silver ion release is sustained over the entire period of application (7 days) provided wound exudate is absorbed into the dressing
- may cause transient discolouration of the wound bed which can be removed by gentle washing
- available as:

CONTREET FOAM
- a silver impregnated polyurethane foam film dressing with and without an adhesive border
- used for medium to heavily exuding chronic wounds

CONTREET FOAM FILLER
- a silver impregnated polyurethane foam film cavity dressing
- used for deep, medium to heavily exuding chronic cavity wounds
- wound is loosely packed to fill approximately half the volume; on absorption of exudate the foam expands and fills the cavity over a short period of time
- not suitable for use on undermined wounds

CONTREET HYDROCOLLOID
- a silver impregnated hydrocolloid/alginate dressing without an adhesive border
- used for low to moderate exuding wounds
- when the exudate reaches the backing film of the dressing, the appearance becomes marbled or transparent

CONVATEC WOUND MANAGER (ConvaTec, DT)
see WOUND DRAINAGE POUCHES
- a wound drainage pouch similar to Biotrol Draina S Fistula and Oakmed Option
- suitable for wounds with a high volume of exudate
- available in three sizes

COSMOPOR E (Hartmann, DT)
see NON/LOW-ADHERENT DRESSINGS (similar to Medipore, Mepore. Primapore, Sterifix)
- absorbent, perforated dressing with a hypoallergenic, adhesive border
- used for post operative wound management and sterile dressings of minor wounds e.g. in first aid

COVERFLEX (Hartmann, DT)
- elasticated Viscose Stockinette
- a lightweight plain-knitted elasticated tubular fabric for dressing retention
- washable for reuse

CRAB COLLAGENASE
- prepared from the hepatopancreas of the king crab (*Paralithodes camtschatica*)

- a comparative study with four other enzyme preparations suggest that crab collagenase is useful in wound debridement[68]

CRYSTAL VIOLET (GENTIAN VIOLET)
see DYES
- in 1987, the DoH advised manufacturers that this should not be used on mucous membranes or open wounds, but should be restricted to topical application on unbroken skin. This was because of reports that systemic absorption of these dyes is carcinogenic in animals

CURAFIL (Tyco Healthcare)
see HYDROGELS
- a hydrogel impregnated gauze dressing containing glycerine
- used for dry to light exuding wounds
- available as pads and a packing strip
- **CURAFIL GEL:** clear wound gel dressing containing glycerine, water and parabens preservatives
- can be used on most wounds except infected wounds and full-thickness burns
- available in various sizes

CURAFOAM ISLAND (Tyco Healthcare, DT)
see FOAMS
- a hydrophilic polyurethane foam film dressing with an adhesive border and a Sontara top sheet
- used for moderate to heavily exuding wounds

CURAFOAM PLUS (Tyco Healthcare, DT)
see FOAMS
- a hydrophilic polyurethane foam film dressing with a blue polyurethane top sheet without an adhesive border
- used for moderate to heavily exuding wounds
- provides a low MVTR, minimising strike through and creates a fluid and bacterial barrier
- applied blue side up and white side to the wound

CURAGEL (Tyco Healthcare, DT)
see HYDROGELS
- a hydrogel dressing available with and without an adhesive border
- consists of polyurethane gel 19%, water 73% and glycol humectant 8%

- used for necrotic wounds, dry to moderate exuding wounds and burns
- maintains balanced hydration through controlled evaporation
- **Curagel** – no adhesive border
- **Curagel Island** – has an adhesive coated polyurethane back sheet and an adhesive border

CURASALT (Tyco Healthcare)
see SODIUM CHLORIDE

- a sponge saturated in a 20% hypertonic saline solution
- used to promote biological cleaning and aid in the autolytic debridement process in infected wounds
- available as a dressing and packing strip

CURASORB (Tyco Healthcare, DT)
see ALGINATES

- a soft, off-white, sterile, non-woven, calcium-sodium alginate dressing available as **Curasorb, Curasorb Plus, Curasorb Zn, Curasorb Rope** and **Curasorb Zn Rope**
- suitable for moderate to heavily exuding wounds, cavity wounds and bleeding wounds
- can absorb 20 times its own weight in exudate (Curasorb Plus even higher)
- forms a gel that remains stable in the presence of exudate
- **Curasorb Zn:** contains less than 1% zinc which helps with cellular mitosis and contributes to cellular proliferation

CURIOSIN (Gideon Richter)
- a 0.2% solution of zinc hyaluronate
- launched in Hungary in 1996
- used for leg ulcers and pressure ulcers

CURITY (Tyco Healthcare)
see NON/LOW ADHERENT DRESSINGS

- a non-adherent dressing consisting of an open mesh, knitted fabric dressing impregnated with an oil emulsion blend
- used for moderate to heavily exuding wounds
- available as strips and dressings

CUTILIN (S & N, DT)
see NON/LOW ADHERENT DRESSINGS

- the shiny contact layer is placed on the wound

CUTINOVA CAVITY
see ALLEVYN PLUS CAVITY

CUTINOVA FOAM
see ALLEVYN COMPRESSION

CUTINOVA HYDRO (S & N, DT)
see HYDROACTIVE DRESSINGS
- polyurethane matrix dressings which does not contain gelling agents
- composed of a polyurethane gel covered with a transparent polyurethane film
- used for light to medium exuding wounds
- dressing change is indicated by a whitish blister in the back of the dressing every 1-3-7 days
- the dressing matrix remains stable when wet, resulting in no leakage, mess and smell
- semi-transparent allowing observation of the wound
- available as square and rectangular dressings:
  Cutinova Hydro: without adhesive border
  Cutinova Hydro Border: absorbent self-adhesive island dressing with adhesive border (formerly known as Cutinova Hydro)

CUTINOVA THIN (Beiersdorf)
see ALLEVYN THIN

C-VIEW (Unomedical, DT)
see VAPOUR-PERMEABLE FILMS
- a vapour-permeable, transparent, self-adhesive film dressing (formerly called Askina Derm)
- consists of a polyurethane film membrane coated with an acrylic adhesive
- may be left in place for up to 7 days

CX POWDER (Adams, DT)
see CHLORHEXIDINE
- a fine powder containing Chlorhexidine acetate 1% w/w in Absorbable Dusting Powder BP
- for general skin disinfection and antisepsis; applied to affected area three times daily
- packaged in a sterile, 15g puffer pack

DAKIN'S SOLUTION (Surgical Chlorinated Soda Solution BPC)
see CHLORINATED SOLUTIONS
- a solution of chlorinated lime, sodium carbonate and boric acid containing 0.5% w/v available chlorine with a pH of 9.5
- first introduced for topical use in open wounds during World War 1 by Nobel Prize winner Alexis Carrel
- needs to be freshly prepared as it is only stable for 2–3 weeks
- not recommended for wound care

DEBRISAN BEADS (Pharmacia)
- hydrophilic, sterile spherical beads of dextranomer (dextran, a carbohydrate polymer cross-linked with epichlorohydrin)
- sprinkle onto wound to a thickness of at least 3mm
- 1g of beads absorb up to 4g of exudate; capillary action carries debris and bacteria away from the wound surface; small molecules enter the beads themselves
- when the beads are fully saturated, the system returns to its original state unless replaced first with new material once or twice a day
- used only on sloughy, exuding wounds and should not be allowed to dry out
- rinsing away the soiled beads can be difficult and uncomfortable (dextranomer is not biodegradable)

DEBRISAN PASTE (Pharmacia)
- a sterile soft, white, granular paste consisting of dextranomer 6.4g, polyethylene glycol 600 and water to 10g
- renew according to the rate of exudation, usually twice daily to every two days
- advised method of application is cumbersome
- Intrasite Gel is more effective at promoting debridement than Debrisan Paste[69]
- Debrisan Paste and Intrasite Gel are both efficacious in the debridement of non-viable tissue. Intrasite Gel had a greater impact in reducing wound area; was superior in ease of application and removal, in reducing pain on application and removal; and in patient comfort during wear[70]

DENIDOR (Jeffreys, Miller)
see DEODORISING DRESSINGS
- activated carbon, deodorising dressing pad
- non-sterile – therefore, do not use as a primary dressing

DEODORISING CARBON DRESSINGS

see ACTISORB SILVER 220, CARBOFLEX, CARBONET, CARBOPAD VC, CLINISORB, DENIDOR, LYOFOAM C (sugar and metronidazole products can also be used to control odour)

- used in the management of discharging, purulent and contaminated wounds complicated by bacterial infection and offensive odour, e.g. fungating carcinomas, leg ulcers, pressure ulcers, gangrenous lesions, etc.
- during their preparation the charcoal fibres become microporous and develop thin, slit-like pores. A high adsorptive performance results from the substantially increased total surface area which is created
- activated charcoal reduces the concentration of offensive odour to low levels
- some dressings adsorb bacteria. The precise method by which bacteria are attracted is not clear, although it has been suggested that there could be an electrostatic or physico-chemical affinity between the charcoal and the bacteria
- some dressings do not maintain a moist environment over the wound, e.g. Actisorb Silver 220, Denidor
- the odour adsorbing capability of five of the dressings has been assessed[71]
- anaerobic bacteria are commonly found in chronic wounds, particularly those that are infected. Several of the Gram-negative anaerobes are the primary causes of wound malodour and consequently their eradication is necessary for the elimination of malodour. Malodour severity may be increased as a consequence of aerobic and anaerobic micro-organisms working in synergy. Disruption of microbial interactions may thus be important in the control of wound malodour[72]

DERMABOND (Ethicon, DT)

see ADHESIVES (TISSUE), EPIGLU, INDERMIL and LIQUIBAND

- sterile tissue adhesive product containing 2-Octyl Cyanoacrylate
- produces similar cosmetic results to suturing but in one third of the time (3.6 minutes vs. 12.4 minutes)
- 2-3 layers of adhesive are applied
- sets in approximately 1 minute and provides the strength of approximated, healed tissue at 7 days, in just 2.5 minutes
- it is not absorbed by skin or underlying tissue;
- used for low tension wounds on scalp, face, trunk and limbs (wounds under tension need to have appropriate subcutaneous sutures placed prior to adhesive application
- there have been no reports of toxicity or carcinogenicity when used topically; there is minimal tissue reaction at 7–14 days
- it sloughs from the wound as re-epithelialisation of skin occurs

48

DERMAFILM (Vygon UK)
see VAPOUR-PERMEABLE FILMS
- self-adhesive, sterile drape for surgery and wound dressings

DERMAGRAFT (Advanced Tissue Sciences in partnership with S & N)
see SKIN SUBSTITUTES
- a human dermal replacement consisting of new-born human fibroblast cells cultured *in vitro* on a bioabsorbable scaffold under aseptic conditions
- the source of the cells are foreskins from circumcised babies. Each foreskin can make more than 23,000 square metres of dermis
- as fibroblasts proliferate within the scaffold, they secrete human dermal collagen, matrix proteins and growth factors to form a human dermal tissue
- used as a permanent replacement dermis that provides a healthy wound bed which promotes epithelialisation, resulting in faster healing of significantly more full-thickness (deep) diabetic foot ulcers that have been present for longer than 6 weeks
- also used for ulcers that extend deeper into the skin where the blood vessels are, but do not involve tendon, muscle, joint capsule or bone
- recommended treatment regimen is one piece implanted in the ulcer weekly, until the ulcer is healed. In a large multicentre controlled study up to eight applications were used. Previously implanted tissue is NOT removed
- no allergic or immunological reactions have been reported to date
- should not be used in patients with known hypersensitivity to bovine serum albumin
- the product is manufactured, frozen and supplied within the protective confines of a bioreactor containing one piece of tissue measuring 5×7.5cm (2×3ins)
- the bioreactor is stored at $-70°C$ and supplied in an insulated container packed with dry ice
- before application, the bioreactor is thawed, opened, and the dermal tissue is rinsed by a medical professional
- the ulcer is traced to allow sizing and shaping of the tissue to fit the wound bed which must meet the criteria for skin grafting
- The York Health Economics Consortium have estimated that at a cost of £250 per piece, Dermagraft is expected to reduce the annual cost per patient treated from £3,620 to £3,492 (a saving of £128 per patient)
- launched in the UK in October 1997 (current cost is £258.75 per piece) and in the USA in 2001

DERMAL PADS (Spenco Healthcare International)
- provide an extra layer of synthetic tissue protection that cushions and protects areas of the body which lack soft tissue padding, e.g. sacrum, heels, elbows
- absorb pressure and will help reduce the effects of both pressure and friction
- will naturally adhere to any skin surface and may be held in place by tape or bandage. They are NOT used as primary wound dressings
- can be easily cut and shaped to fit requirements and are re-usable

DESLOUGHERS AND CLEANSERS
see ASERBINE, CHLORAMINE, CHLORINATED SOLUTIONS, DAKIN'S, DEBRISAN, EUSOL, GRANUGEL, HIOXYL, HYDROCOLLOIDS, HYDROGEN PEROXIDE, INTRASITE GEL, IODOFLEX, IODOSORB, MILTON, NORMASOL, SODIUM CHLORIDE, SUGAR PASTE, VARIDASE[73]
- there is insufficient evidence to promote the use of one debriding agent over another[74]
- there is only a single comparison between two debriding agents that produced a significant result – Intrasite Gel significantly reduced necrotic wound area compared with dextranomer polysaccharide paste[69]
- a review is available of NICE guidance on the use of debriding agents and specialist wound care clinics for difficult to heal surgical wounds[75]

DRESSINGS (GENERAL)[76, 77]
- the Isle of Wight PCT has piloted a novel scheme for the supply of dressings. The scheme removes the need for GPs or nurse prescriptions and allows nurses to order dressings in larger amounts rather than for individual patients. The scheme reduces waste, cost and time spent prescribing and dispensing dressings[78]
- the supply of the first dressing for the patient is often delayed by obtaining a prescription. To avoid this, Stockport PCT have implemented a scheme to supply nurses with wound dressing starter packs[79]

DRESS-IT (Richardson Healthcare, DT)
- a non Drug Tariff specification sterile dressing pack containing:
    - 1 paper towel
    - 1 disposable bag
    - 4 softswabs 12 ply
    - 1 dressing pad
    - 1 softdrape

DRISORB (Vernon-Carus, DT)
see NON/LOW-ADHERENT DRESSINGS
- low-adherent, absorbent dressing pad
- used as a secondary dressing in conjunction with a primary wound dressing

DUODERM
see GRANUFLEX, HYDROCOLLOIDS
- American/European form of Granuflex
- the Duoderm hydrocolloid dressings possess effective physical barrier properties to both HIV-1 and Hepatitis B virus when stringently challenged *in vitro*[80]

DUODERM EXTRA THIN (ConvaTec, DT)
see GRANUFLEX and HYDROCOLLOIDS
- thin, semi-permeable hydrocolloid dressing without adhesive border (formerly Granuflex Extra Thin)
- consists of an inner layer of hydrocolloids contained within an adhesive polymer matrix and an outer layer of polyurethane film
- used for acute and chronic lightly exuding wounds, e.g. post-operative sutured wounds, superficial pressure ulcers, abrasions
- particularly suitable in areas where movement is necessary because the dressing is highly flexible
- should not be left in place for longer than 7 days

DUODERM SIGNAL (ConvaTec, DT)
see HYDROCOLLOIDS
- a hydrocolloid dressing with tapered border edges similar to Comfeel Bevelled Edge Dressing
- used on acute and chronic wounds
- flexible and conformable
- translucent enabling visual access to the wound
- as dressing absorbs exudate, it forms a gel that may be visible as a bubble underneath the surface of the dressing. If the bubble expands to any part of the dotted dressing-change indicator line, the dressing should be changed to avoid leakage. Dressing should be used up to a maximum of 7 days
- available as square, heel and sacral shapes for hard to dress areas

DURASIS (Cook)
see SKIN SUBSTITUTES and SURGISIS
- used as a dural substitute for repairing dura mater

DYES

- can be divided into five groups, the two main types being the acridine and triphenyl-methane derivatives which are bacteriostatic:
  1. Acridines e.g. acriflavine, proflavine
  2. Eosin 2% w/v – popular in Scotland
  3. Mercurochrome 1–2%
  4. Potassium permanganate 1:8000 to 1:10,000 e.g. Permitabs
  5. Triphenyl methanes e.g. brilliant green 0.5%; crystal violet (gentian violet) 0.5%; magenta; malachite green
- traditionally used for their antimicrobial activity and as astringents to dry up macerated skin around wounds
- modern use has declined because of the lack of information on their clinical effectiveness and fears about their detrimental effects on wound healing

EASI-V (Unomedical)
see VAPOUR-PERMEABLE FILMS
- sterile semi-permeable adhesive film with foam border
- used as a securement device for I.V. peripheral lines
- helps to prevent the ingress of secretions and micro-organisms, thus reducing infections
- can be used for up to 5 days

ECLYPSE (Advancis Medical, DT)
- a highly absorptive wound exudate dressing
- absorbent cellulose dressing with a fluid repellent backing consisting of:
  - a rapid wicking polyester and viscose woven wound contact layer
  - layer of mechanically bonded cellulose
  - a strong, polyester, fluid repellent blue backing
- used for medium to heavily exuding wounds
- avoid using on any arterial bleeds or heavily bleeding wounds
- dressings can be placed side-by-side to cover large wound areas
- initially may need frequent changes but can be left in place for up to 7 days depending on exudate levels

EGG PRODUCTS
- the use of egg white has been specifically prohibited by the Department of Health since 1988. "Some nurses and midwives continue to use raw eggs on pressure sores, ulcers and babies' sore bottoms. SUCH PRACTICES SHOULD CEASE IMMEDIATELY"[81]

ENSURE-IT (Becton Dickinson)
see VAPOUR-PERMEABLE FILMS

EOSIN
see DYES
- 2% w/v aqueous eosin paint; a colouring agent
- bacteriostatic and fungistatic solution with a very broad spectrum; Pseudomonas is not sensitive
- dries up the granulation edges of a wound if it is too liberally applied

EPI-FIX (Unomedical)
see VAPOUR-PERMEABLE FILMS
- for fixation of epidural catheters
- can be used for up to 5 days

EPIGLU (ICN Pharmaceuticals Ltd, DT)
see ADHESIVES (TISSUE), DERMABOND, INDERMIL AND LIQUIBAND
- contains ethyl-2-cyanoacrylate and polymethylmethacrylate
- used as a tissue adhesive for external use to fresh incisions and lacerations (also post-operative), closure of wounds (after careful adaption of the wound edges) and as a suture substitute or for additional suture support
- should be used by trained medical staff only
- seal the closed wound edges, either by dabs of Epiglu or by lightly covering the entire wound. Epiglu adheres within seconds and subsequent correction is not possible. After the first application has hardened, apply a second, slightly wider layer and allow to set. Repeat procedure if required, allowing each layer to set for approximately 2 minutes
- very rarely, an allergic reaction may occur
- available as vials containing approximately 20 applications
- should be stored in the refrigerator or freezer and can be used immediately without requiring warming up
- available as 4 vials containing 80 applications

ESSENTIAL OILS[82]
- Ylang Ylang, Wintergreen: in the management of pain
- Bergamot, St. John's Wort: in the management of odour
- St John's Wort, German chamomile: to promote granulation tissue
- Lavender, Roman chamomile: as an inflammatory agent
- Myrrh, Tea Tree: for wound cleaning

ETE (Mölnlycke)
see NON/LOW ADHERENT DRESSINGS
- pad of rayon wadding with rayon silk wound contact layer stitched in chequered pattern; apply shiny side to the wound

EUSOL
see CHLORINATED SOLUTIONS[83]
- Edinburgh University SOlution of Lime: solution of chlorinated lime and boric acid containing not less than 0.25% w/v available chlorine with a pH of 7.5–8.5
- used for infected, necrotic ulcers; has an effective action against bacteria such as staphylococcus and pseudomonas
- must be freshly prepared and has a two-week expiry
- there is a rapid inactivation of the antiseptic effect when contaminated by organic materials, e.g. pus and dressings
- caustic to ulcer and surrounding skin; destroys and damages healing tissue
- may cause the release of endotoxins from micro-organisms, e.g. coliforms. This may cause side effects ranging from mild uraemic toxaemia to serious renal failure (Schwartzmann reaction)
- may cause the formation of exuberant and excessive granulation tissue
- the addition of paraffin prevents dressing adherence and maintains a moist environment e.g. Eusol and Liquid Paraffin Emulsion
- Eusol, half-strength Eusol and Eusol and Liquid Paraffin Emulsion should not be used for wound care – disadvantages outweigh the benefits
- alternative agents are listed in the section on Management of wounds/wound types

EXU-DRY (S & N, DT)
see NON/LOW ADHERENT DRESSING
- an absorbent cellulose dressing with a fluid repellent backing (similar to Mesorb)
- a multi-layered dressing consisting of:
  - a low adherent wound contact layer
  - an anti-shear layer to reduce pain and trauma
  - highly absorbent inner layers
  - semi-permeable outer layer
- can be used as a primary or secondary dressing for medium to heavily exuding wounds

FLAMAZINE (S & N, POM)
see ANTIBACTERIALS and SILVER

- a hydrophilic cream containing silver sulfadiazine 1% w/w oil-in-water emulsion; also contains polysorbates, glycerol monoester, cetyl alcohol, liquid paraffin, propylene glycol and purified water
- combines the antiseptic properties of silver with the antibacterial properties of sulphonamide
- topical broad-spectrum antibacterial; inhibits the growth of nearly all pathogenic bacteria and fungi in vitro
- used to treat a variety of wounds where infection may prevent healing e.g. leg ulcers, pressure ulcers, burns etc.
- marked antibacterial action against MRSA – 51 strains (100% effective), gentamicin-resistant pseudomonas (21 strains), gentamicin-resistant enterococci – (23 strains) and glycopeptide-resistant enterococci (54 strains)
- has achieved wide acceptance as the agent of choice for the prevention of Gram-negative sepsis in patients with extensive burns (first used in burns in 1968)
- antibacterial activity is prolonged because of the gradual release of silver ions which act on the bacterial cell surface to cause drastic alterations in the cell wall and plasma membrane
- mainly used under absorbent dressings which are changed daily (for burns) or at least three times a week (for leg ulcers)
- leucopenia has been reported in 3–5% of burns patients treated with cream
- sensitivity reactions occur uncommonly but the incidence is lower than with other sulphonamides; the vast majority of sensitisation reactions are due to one of the excipients in the cream
- the emergence of silver resistant bacteria has been reported
- use with caution if renal/hepatic function becomes impaired
- argyria has been reported[84] with excessive use (50g every 2 days for 5 months)
- cream should not be applied to skin surrounding the ulcer otherwise it may cause maceration
- in a prospective randomised trial, Mepitel reduces healing time in burned paediatric patients in comparison with silver sulfadiazine treatment[85]
- Now included in the list of preparations which may be prescribed by Extended Formulary Nurse Prescribers. It is used in the prevention of Gram-negative sepsis in patients with extensive burns. It is also used on infected leg ulcers and pressure ulcers.

FLEXI-BAN (Activa Health Care, DT)
- sub-compression wadding bandage

FLEXIPORE (Innovative Technologies, DT)
see FOAMS (formerly known as Spyroflex and Cliniflex)
- sterile, vapour-permeable dressing consisting of two layers:
  - pressure-sensitive hydrophilic adhesive
  - flexible microporous polyurethane membrane
- gas/moisture vapour permeable, yet provides an effective barrier to water/bacteria
- used for lightly exuding wounds, including minor trauma
- not recommended for use on grossly infected wounds
- should be changed on exuding wounds after seven days
- may be cut/overlapped if necessary
- manufactured by Innovative Technologies and distributed by Tissue Science Laboratories, Greyholme House, 49 Victoria Road, Aldershot, Hampshire GU11 1SJ

FOAM DRESSINGS
see 3M FOAM, ACTIVHEAL, ADVAZORB, ALLEVYN RANGE, AVANCE RANGE, BIATAIN, CAVI-CARE, CONTREET, CURAFOAM, FLEXIPORE, HYDRAFOAM, LYOFOAM, LYOSHEET, PERMAFOAM, TIELLE, TRANSORBENT, TRUFOAM
- consist of absorbent polyurethane and other components:
  - hydrocellular foams (multi-layered)
  - hydropolymer foams (multi-layered)
  - soft silicone foams (Mepiform, Mepilex)
  - foam plus silver (Avance, Contreet)
  - foam plus carbon (Lyofoam C)
- suitable for flat and cavity wounds with a varying amount of exudate
- not suitable for the management of dry necrotic wounds except in conjunction with a suitable debriding agent
- the correct surface should be applied to the wound
- characteristics of a good foam product are good adhesion and fluid handling capacity (a combination of moisture vapour transmission rate and absorbance); this will reduce the number of dressing changes
- available in either flat sheets (with or without an adhesive border) or as a cavity dressing

FUCIDIN (Leo, DT, POM)
see ANTIBIOTICS
- cream contains fusidic acid 2%
- ointment contains sodium fusidate 2% and wool fat
- topical use carries the risk of skin sensitisation
- not recommended for wound care

GEL FX (Vernon-Carus, DT)
see HYDROGELS
- a hydrogel coated polyester net with large perforations
- the hydrogel contains approximately 30% water; the remaining 70% consists of a partially swollen crosslinked polymer network and humectant
- used as a primary dressing for the treatment of burns, nail avulsions, skin tears and leg ulcers
- used in conjunction with an absorbent secondary dressing which is changed leaving Gel FX in place
- the large perforations allow the passage of exudate from the wound into the secondary dressing
- available in square and rectangular sizes

GELIPERM (Geistlich Pharma, DT)
see HYDROGELS
- available as a wet sheet (without adhesive border) containing 96% water and a mixture of 1% agar and 3% polyacrylamide
- impermeable to bacteria but permeable to water vapour and gases
- absorbent and may be used on lightly exuding wounds or dry wounds
- feels wet and cold on touch but is neither
- transparent so wound can be inspected if exudate is clear
- sometimes during application it becomes dry and brittle on a wound because of evaporation; rehydration may be necessary. It is a difficult dressing to handle
- on average needs changing every 3-4 days. Heavily exuding wounds may require to be changed daily. The dressing needs changing when it has become cloudy or opaque due to the absorption of wound exudate
- the results of a laboratory study suggest that Geliperm (and Vigilon) are likely to be ideally suited only to wounds that exude at a rate which is compatible with the fluid handling properties of the dressings[86]

GRANEODIN (Squibb, POM, DT)

see ANTIBIOTICS

- ointment containing 0.25% neomycin and 0.025% gramicidin in Plastibase
- applied 2–4 times daily for a maximum of 7 days
- sensitivity to neomycin and gramicidin may occur
- ototoxicity and nephrotoxicity have been reported
- not recommended for wound care

GRANUFLEX (Convatec, DT)

see HYDROCOLLOIDS

- consists of an outer waterproof polyurethane foam, bonded onto a polyurethane film, which acts as a carrier for the hydrocolloid base. The base consists of gelatin, pectin, carboxymethylcellulose, adhesives and other polymers
- the hydrocolloids are held in a matrix which is cross-linked and this forms a stable mass in which the gel is contained
- used for light to medium exuding wounds
- dependent on exudate, the dressing can be left in place for up to seven days
- available as bordered and non-bordered dressings including triangular shapes which are specially designed to fit sacral pressure ulcers
- the hypoxic and acidic environment under the dressings encourages angiogenesis resulting in the development of healthy granulation tissue
- there is published evidence of resolution and prevention of fibrin clots under Granuflex
- Comfeel and Granuflex have been compared[55]
- in a randomised controlled clinical study comparing Tielle with Granuflex, Tielle was better in preventing leakage and reducing odour, but there were no differences in healing rates of patients with leg ulcers or pressure ulcers[87]
- in a randomised comparison comparing Allevyn Adhesive with Granuflex, the data indicate that both dressings are easy and convenient to apply; absorbency and ease of removal were better with Allevyn; wear times were similar[20]
- the results from a European study show Granuflex to be 50% more cost-effective, at £422 per healed wound, than Comfeel (£643) and 500% more so than saline gauze (£2548) in the treatment of pressure sores. Granuflex at £342 was also more cost-effective than gauze (£541) or Apligraf (£6741) in the treatment of venous leg ulcers[88]
- a chronic inflammatory reaction has been reported in full-thickness excised lesions on porcine skin. This appeared to be in response to particulate matter that had been incorporated into the wound bed and hypodermis, and was still apparent six months after injury, when hydrocolloid particles were detectable microscopically in the hypodermis[89]. A subsequent histological evaluation of

chronic human wounds treated with hydrocolloid and non-hydrocolloid dressings showed no significant adverse histological sequelae[90]
- **GRANUFLEX Paste:** for cavity wounds
- **GRANUFLEX Bordered:** consists of an adhesive polyurethane foam which extends 2.0–2.5cm around area of hydrocolloid; specifically designed to fit sacral and difficult to dress areas

GRANUGEL (ConvaTec, DT)
see, HYDROCOLLOIDS and HYDROGELS
- a sterile, smooth, clear gel containing hydrocolloid powders. The gel consists of 80% water with sodium carboxymethylcellulose, pectin and propylene glycol (15%)
- gel is viscous with a slight adhesive tack allowing easy application
- indicated for deep and superficial wounds, dry, sloughy and necrotic wounds
- in dry conditions, the gel releases moisture, thus aiding the natural autolytic process. On moist wounds, the gel is capable of absorbing twice its weight in fluid
- gel is changed at intervals not exceeding three days when used on sloughy, necrotic wounds, or seven days on clean granulating wounds
- available in 15g single use tubes with sterile nozzle

GROWTH FACTORS (chemical messengers)
see REGRANEX
- also known as Colony-Stimulating Factors, Cytokines and Interleukins
- includes cytokines and peptides of low molecular weight which act locally, having a specific high affinity for cell surface receptors and the ability to stimulate or inhibit cell proliferation or differentiation[91, 92, 93]
- small amounts originally available from natural sources; recombinant growth factors are now produced in large amounts by the biotechnology industry
- over 30 growth factors (GFs) have been identified of three main types: proliferative (causing cell replication), migratory (chemoattractants which stimulate movement of cells) and transforming which produce a phenotypic alteration[94, 95]:
  - Epidermal GFs:
    - EGF: Epidermal GF (epithelialisation)
    - TGF-alpha: Transforming GF alpha (epithelialisation)
    - Heparin-binding epidermal GF
  - Fibroblast GFs:
    - FGF-2: Basic Fibroblast GF (angiogenesis and fibroblast proliferation)

- FGF-1: Acidic Fibroblast GF (angiogenesis and fibroblast proliferation)
- KGF: Keratinocyte GF: (epidermal cell motiliy and proliferation)
- Transforming GFs:
  - TGF-beta: Transforming GF beta (matrix synthesis, inhibitor of proliferation
- Other GFs:
  - PDGF: Platelet-derived GF (angiogenesis, fibroplasia)
  - VEGF: Vascular endothelial GF (angiogenesis)
  - Tumour necrosis GF alpha
  - 1L–1: Interleukin–1 (inflammatory cell recruitment, matrix synthesis)
  - ILG–1: Insulin-like GF 1 (fibroplasia)
  - M–CSF: Monocyte-colony stimulating GF (monocyte migration and maturation)
  - GM–CSF: Granulocyte monocyte-colony stimulating GF (monocyte migration and maturation)
  - CTGF: Connective Tissue Growth Factor (proliferation, matrix synthesis)
- currently only one growth factor is available commercially – Regranex
- clinical studies in the treatment of non-healing human wounds have reported disappointing results. GFs are destroyed by protein-degrading enzymes in the wound[96]
- further work needs to be carried out to determine which growth factors are appropriate for each type of chronic wound and in what combinations[97]

H–F ANTIDOTE GEL (IPS Health Care)
- contains Calcium Gluconate BP 2.5% in a clear, water-miscible gel base
- used as first-aid treatment of hydrofluoric acid burns to reduce burn damage to bone and deep tissue
- calcium gluconate combines with hydrofluoric acid to neutralise the fluoride ion
- available as a kit containing 3 × 25g tubes of gel, gloves and guidance card (£44.93 + VAT)

HAEMOSTATICS
see ALGINATES, OXYCEL and SURGICEL
- compounds used for the treatment or prophylaxis of haemorrhage by inhibiting the breakdown of the fibrin clot
- oxidised cellulose is an absorbable haemostatic which should not be used as a surface dressing, except for immediate control of bleeding as it inhibits epithelialisation
- some alginates are ideal for bleeding wounds

HAIR REMOVERS

- depilatory creams should be used rather than shaving which "nicks" the skin and may cause infection

HIOXYL CREAM (Ferndale)

see HYDROGEN PEROXIDE SOLUTION

- a white, non-greasy cream containing stabilised hydrogen peroxide, 1.5% (equivalent to 5 volume hydrogen peroxide) of low pH
- gives a prolonged antiseptic action (for at least eight hours) which is a result of its steady release of oxygen when applied to tissues
- clinical experience indicates that the optimal dressing frequency for a sloughy wound is daily. Once cleansing has been established, application every other day or even every third day has been found to be acceptable
- may sting when applied
- do not mix with other topical medicaments likely to react with hydrogen peroxide

HONEY[98, 99]

see ACTIVON TULLE, API-BAN, HONEY (ANTIBACTERIAL), HONEYSOFT, SUGAR

- has been used in wound care since the time of the Ancient Egyptians when it was the most popular drug
- the development of wound care products containing honey has been limited by the availability of standardised, quality assured preparations, although the situation is changing[100]
- contains digested sugars (glucose and fructose), vitamins, minerals and enzymes
- will not support bacteria growth because of its high osmotic pressure
- antibacterial activity is due mainly to hydrogen peroxide which is liberated by an enzyme reaction. Some types of honey may also contain antibacterial substances derived from flowers visited by bees[101]
- has effective antibacterial, debriding and anti-inflammatory properties; acts as a stimulant for the growth of new blood capillaries, fibroblasts and epithelial cells[102, 103]
- randomised controlled trials have shown that in honey-dressed wounds, early subsidence of acute inflammatory changes, better control of infection and quicker wound healing was observed compared to silver sulphadiazine in controlling infection in burn wounds[104]

- honeys with an average level of antibacterial activity could be expected to be effective in preventing the growth of pseudomonads on the surface of a wound even if the honey were diluted more than ten-fold by exudation from the wound[105]
- it is progressively diluted with exudate during use. This reduces its osmotic effect but other antimicrobial components in honey will ensure that inhibition is maintained[106]
- honey is a viscous liquid which is difficult to retain in the wound; dressing pads pre-impregnated with honey are the most convenient method of applying honey to wounds (rather than directly to the wound)
- for wound care, large amounts of honey should be applied to maintain potency
- it is non-irritant and has a low pH
- do not use in diabetics: glucose and fructose can be absorbed from an open wound
- adverse reactions are rare but may be caused by reaction to a specific pollen in the honey. Localised stinging may be due to the acidity of honey
- researchers at the University of Wales Institute are conducting trials on the use of absorbent pads impregnated with active Manuka honey from New Zealand. The dressings are irradiated and used to treat recurrent wound infections
- is prone to contamination with clostridial spores and non-pathogenic *Bacillus* spp.
- honey for clinical uses should be sterile and derived from specified pathogen-free hives, which have not been treated with drugs, and are gathered in areas where no pesticides are used[107]
- two types of honey and an artificial honey solution were assessed to determine how effectively they inhibited antibiotic-resistant and antibiotic-sensitive bacteria that could cause wound infections. Both types of natural honey were found to be effective at inhibiting bacteria, including antibiotic-resistant bacteria. The artificial honey solution needed to be three times the concentration of the natural honeys to produce the same inhibitory effects. The inhibition of bacteria by honey is not exclusively due to osmolarity. A possible role for honey in the treatment of wounds colonised by antibiotic-resistant bacteria is indicated[108]
- All you ever wanted to know about honey –
see www.archive.uwcm.ac.uk/uwcm/sr/whru/Honey.html

HONEY, ANTIBACTERIAL (Medihoney)
see API-BAN and HONEY
- pure honey derived from selected *Leptospermum* spp.

- particularly effective against *Staphylococcus aureus* and *Pseudomonas* spp.
- available in 50g tubes
- further information is available at: www.medihoney.com

HONEYSOFT (Euro Surgical Ltd)
see HONEY DRESSINGS

- consists of ethylenenvinylacetate (a low-adherent material) impregnated with medicinal honey free of pollutants such as pesticides and heavy metals
- contains glucose oxidase which ensures continuous release of hydrogen peroxide in non-toxic low doses; this provides anti-bacterial protection of the wound
- a secondary dressing is needed
- preferably change every 24 hours
- 2 sterile sizes available

HORMONE REPLACEMENT THERAPY (HRT)
- oestrogens are known to have an effect on skin and other soft tissues
- case-cohort studies have shown that HRT users over 65 are about 30-40% less likely to develop a venous leg ulcer or pressure ulcer than non-users. This may be evidence for a preventative effect for HRT on chronic wounds[109]

HOSPI-FOUR (Millpledge Healthcare, DT)
see COMPRESSION BANDAGES (FOUR-LAYER)

HYALOFILL (ConvaTec)
see HYALURONIC ACID

- composed of sterile 100% Hyaff (a biocompatible derivative of hyaluronic acid)
- on contact with wound exudate, completely dissolves to form a thick hyaluronic acid-rich gel which promotes moist wound healing
- used for chronic wound management to promote granulation and contraction in recalcitrant wounds
- used until a healthy granulating wound bed has formed; once this phase has been initiated, moist wound dressings are used to complete wound closure
- depending on the level of exudate, lasts for up to 3 days
- can be cut without linting and can be folded to conform to the wound
- requires a secondary dressing
- 100% biodegradable – Hyaff is broken down to hyaluronic acid and benzyl alcohol which is metabolised and excreted in the urine

- available as fibrous sheets (10 × 10cm, 5 × 5cm)
- **HYALOFILL-R:** absorbent fibrous rope (0.5g)

HYALURONIC ACID
see HYALOFILL and SEPRAFILM
- a major carbohydrate component of the extracellular matrix of skin, joints, eyes and most organs and tissues
- can absorb up to 3000 times its own weight in water
- accelerates tissue repair by:
  - inducing a prompt angiogenic response
  - regulation of inflammation
  - prompting rapid formation of granulation tissue
  - assisting fibroblast growth and movement
  - directing the organisation of collagen deposition

HYDRAFOAM (Tyco Healthcare, DT)
see FOAMS
- a hydrophilic, polyurethane foam film dressing without an adhesive border
- used for moderate to heavily exuding wounds
- non-sided (each side has same composition and characteristics)

HYDROACTIVE DRESSINGS
see ALLEVYN range and CUTINOVA HYDRO
- manufactured from polyurethane matrix containing super-absorbent molecules
- selectively absorbs mainly water, leaving essential ingredients for wound healing on the wound bed (physiological cleansing of wound)
- used on exuding wounds from deep cavities to skin graft donor sites
- do not require secondary dressings
- does not adhere to wound bed
- no gel residue is left on wound bed, lessening the need for intensive irrigation
- recommended that dressings are changed within 2–3 days or sooner, depending on level of exudate. As healing proceeds, frequency of dressing change reduces
- remains stable when wet, making dressings easy to handle at dressing change
- molecular structure prevents squeeze out under compression
- some patients experience tingling sensation due to physiological debriding action

HYDROCOLL (Hartmann, DT)
see HYDROCOLLOIDS
- self-adhesive, absorbent hydrocolloid dressing covered with a semi-permeable polyurethane layer

- improved formulation does not contain gelatin or other animal derivatives known to cause allergic reactions
- suitable for light to medium exuding wounds
- available in the Drug Tariff in a variety of sizes and shapes including presentations with bevelled edges to fit heels, elbows and sacral areas:
  - **Hydrocoll basic**
  - **Hydrocoll** – with bevelled edges
  - **Hydrocoll thin**
  - **Hydrocoll sacral** – shaped dressing with bevelled edges and flexible hinge
  - **Hydrocoll heel/elbow** – shaped dressing with bevelled edges
  - **Hydrocoll Border (bevelled edge):** concave dressing

HYDROCOLLOIDS
see ACTIVHEAL, ALIONE, AQUACEL, ASKINA BIOFILM TRANSPARENT, COMBIDERM, COMFEEL, COMPEED HYDRO CURE, CONTREET, CUTINOVA, DUODERM, GRANUFLEX, GRANUGEL, HYDROCOLL, REPLICARE ULTRA, SEASORB SOFT, SUPRASORB H, TEGASORB, ULTEC PRO, URGOSORB, URGOTUL, VARIHESIVE, VERSIVA[55, 110, 111]

- a hydrocolloid is a microgranular suspension of various natural or synthetic polymers, e.g. gelatin or pectin, in an adhesive matrix, e.g. polyisobutylene, the granules being in a semi-hydrated state and hydrophilic, and the adhesive matrix being of a hydrophobic nature. Standardisation of constituents may be a problem
- dressings should extend at least 2cm beyond the edge of the wound
- may release degradation products from the dressing into the wound[89]
- dressings are "interactive" in contact with wound exudate. Hydrocolloids slowly absorb fluid leading to a change in the physical state of the dressing, forming a gel which may be cohesive and/or hydrophilic; some products retain the resultant gel within its cross-linked matrix
- provide an environment conducive to rapid debridement, thus there may be an initial increase in wound size
- when the hydrocolloid liquifies, it swells into the cavity and applies pressure to the base of the wound
- suitable for desloughing and for light to medium exuding wounds
- the manufacturers' recommendations should be followed when treating infected wounds. In a prospective trial, the risk of clinical infection is less under occlusive dressings such as hydrocolloids than under conventional impregnated gauze dressings (tulle gras) in small partial thickness burns,

donor sites and venous leg ulcers[112]. A retrospective review shows similar results[113]
- the use of hydrocolloids in the treatment of diabetic foot wounds has been reviewed[114]
- require no secondary dressing
- initially may need changing daily. Once the exudate has diminished, dressings may be left in place for up to seven days. Heavy exudate leads to too frequent changes of dressing
- dressings promote the formation of granulation tissue
- provide pain relief by keeping nerve endings moist
- in an *in vitro* assay, the hydrophilic particles of five hydrocolloid dressings significantly inhibited fibroblast proliferation[115]
- have barrier properties of varying degrees to gases, moisture vapour and micro-organisms
- are variably transparent/semi-transparent in use
- waterproof, so patient can bath or shower; the dressing should seal round the borders of a wound
- odour may be a concern with some dressings and patients should be informed beforehand
- hydrocolloids have many of the characteristics of an ideal dressing (*see* appendix)
- available in different forms with different properties – wafers (thick and thin), granules, powders, gels and paste

HYDROFILM (Hartmann, DT)
see VAPOUR-PERMEABLE FILMS

HYDROGELS
see ACTIFORMCOOL, ACTIVHEAL, AQUAFLO, AQUAFORM, CLEARSITE, CURAFIL, CURAGEL, GEL FX, GELIPERM, GRANUGEL, HYDROSORB, HYPERGEL, INTRASITE, MOTHERMATES, NORMLGEL, NOVOGEL, NU-GEL, OPRAGEL, PRIMSKIN, PURILON, SUPRASORB G
- available as flat sheets or amorphous gels having a high water content – gels are more commonly used
- hydrogels with a high water content can rehydrate wounds and ensure moist wound healing
- cool the surface of the wound – this is said to be the cause of the marked reduction in pain. Products can be refrigerated to increase this effect
- suitable for desloughing and for light to medium exuding wounds
- can be left on the wound for variable times – 1–5 days

- care must be taken to apply the correct amount of hydrogel - too much will cause maceration of the skin and wound
- should not be used on highly exuding wounds as this will cause maceration
- contra-indicated where anaerobic infection is suspected – can support the growth of micro-organisms
- have a favourable permeability profile for gases
- some can act as a carrier for water soluble, topical medicaments
- some allow monitoring of the wound without disturbing the dressing
- sheet hydrogels may be used "cut-to-shape" of the wound or may overlap
- they do not swell into a wound like the hydrocolloids
- most hydrogels need a secondary dressing
- the results of a laboratory study suggest that Geliperm and Vigilon are likely to be ideally suited only to wounds that exude at a rate which is compatible with the fluid handling properties of the dressings[86]
- hydrogels have many of the characteristics of an ideal dressing (*see* appendix) but there may be some difficulties in application

HYDROGEN PEROXIDE SOLUTION
see HIOXL

- usual strength of solution is 10 volume (3%)
- caustic effect on wounds in concentrations above 20 volume (6%)
- used to clean dirty, infected, necrotic, sloughy wounds but is not recommended on clean wounds
- contamination with organic material results in loss of effectiveness
- has an antiseptic effect due to its release of oxygen when applied to tissues – 1ml hydrogen peroxide 3% (10 volume) will release 10ml oxygen (oxidising agent)
- reacts with catalase causing frothing which helps to lift out foreign matter from the wound
- beware chemical interactions with other agents
- irrigation of hydrogen peroxide solution under pressure or into enclosed body cavities may have serious consequences such as oxygen embolus and surgical emphysema[116]. A patient died due to air embolism attributed to hydrogen peroxide[117]
- may be caustic to surrounding skin and wound[23, 118]
- at low concentrations, may stimulate fibroblast proliferation[119]. At concentrations recommended for wound cleansing, it produced 100% killing of all cell types[53]. Hydrogen peroxide fibroblast toxicity exceeds bacterial toxicity[23]. In an *in vitro* study, at concentrations that preserve fibroblast function, 0.003% hydrogen peroxide solution failed to reduce any bacterial counts[120]

- at present there seems to be insufficient evidence to base definitive judgements about the merits of hydrogen peroxide on wound healing[121]

HYDROSORB (Hartmann)
see HYDROGELS
- a sterile, transparent, self-adhesive hydrogel dressing consisting of 60% water and absorbent polyurethane polymers covered with a semi-permeable polyurethane film (without adhesive border)
- used for the treatment of slow-healing wounds, second-degree burns, abrasions and painful tissue injuries
- the upper surface of the dressing is marked with a grid to aid documentation of wound size
- the three-dimensional gel structure is not dissolved by absorbing wound exudate and thus can be removed from the wound in one piece without leaving any residue
- the gel has a slight cooling effect
- can stay on the wound for up to 7 days
- **HYDROSORB COMFORT** has an additional hypoallergenic, broad, continuous adhesive border to ensure that the dressing stays in place; available in three sizes (square and rectangular)

HYPAFIX (S & N, DT)
- a permeable, apertured non-woven synthetic adhesive tape similar to Mefix

HYPERGEL (Mölnlycke)
see HYDROGELS
- 20% sodium chloride gel which hydrates and draws fluid from the wound
- used on dry necrosis

INADINE (J & J, DT)
see ANTISEPTICS, POVIDERM and POVIDONE-IODINE
- a sterile, low-adherent knitted viscous dressing impregnated with 10% povidone-iodine in a water-soluble polyethylene glycol base
- has been improved by increasing the loading of povidone iodine ointment and by reducing the number of threads
- dressing is now softer and more conformable
- may be used for prophylaxis and treatment of a wide range of bacterial, protozoal and fungal organisms in superficial burns and skin loss injuries
- the dressing should only be changed when the distinctive orange-brown colour changes to white; this indicates that the povidone-iodine has been used up

- the amount of free iodine available is very low but there may be some sensitivity to povidone-iodine or iodine
- not more than four dressings should be used at the same time
- BNF considers this product to be less suitable for prescribing

INDERMIL (Sherwood, Davis & Geck, DT)
see ADHESIVES (TISSUE), DERMABOND, EPIGLU, LIQUIBAND
- sterile tissue adhesive product containing N-butyl cyanoacrylate
- used for low tension wounds on scalp, face, trunk and limbs (wounds under tension need to have appropriate subcutaneous sutures placed prior to adhesive application
- cannula applicator available
- available as a unit dose (0.5g, DT) and clinic kits (5g)

INSULIN
- topical insulin is effective in accelerating the healing of wounds in humans[122]
- this may be due to the insulin and/or to the zinc which it contains

INTEGRA (Integra NeuroSciences)
see SKIN SUBSTITUTES
- is a dermal regeneration template used to treat scars in plastic surgery
- it is an alternative to full-thickness skin grafting, skin expansion and even skin flaps for reconstructive surgery
- the template consists of:
  - a silicone layer which provides immediate wound closure
  - a three dimensional collagen-glycosaminoglycan matrix that serves as a scaffold for dermal regeneration. This promotes cellular ingrowth and initiates regeneration of autologous tissue, which leads to functional new dermis
- as healing progresses, collagen is deposited by fibroblasts, gradually replacing the collagen and glycosaminoglycan layer of the template
- as soon as the neodermis is formed and has been sufficiently vascularised (day 21 onwards after application), the silicone layer can be removed
- the template is incorporated without rejection, biodegraded, leaving autologous dermis in place
- the neodermis is covered with a thin epidermal split thickness graft
- at around day 30, the skin is regenerated with complete wound closure
- Integra restores functionality, improves the visual appearance (compared to meshed split-thickness skin) and gives a low rate of contracture recurrence

- Integra is expensive ranging in price from £547–£1676 per sheet plus £30 carriage

INTERPOSE (Frontier Multigate, DT)
see NON/LOW ADHERENT DRESSING
- range of absorbent, perforated plastic film faced dressing pads available

INTRASITE CONFORMABLE (S & N, DT)
see HYDROGELS and INTRASITE
- a non-woven dressing impregnated with Intrasite Gel
- used for dry, sloughy or necrotic wounds; lightly exuding wounds; granulating wounds
- facilitates the gentle packing of shallow or deep, awkwardly shaped or undetermined wounds
- secondary dressings are required
- range of product sizes available suitable for all wound sizes:
  - 10 × 10cm (7.5g loading)
  - 10 × 20cm (15g loading)
  - 10 × 40cm (30g loading)

INTRASITE GEL (S & N, DT)
see HYDROGELS; formerly known as Scherisorb
- 2.3% modified sodium carboxymethylcellulose (cross-linked) polymer, 77.7% water and 20% propylene glycol (humectant and preservative)
- cross-linked polymer helps the gel to remain in place in the presence of exudate
- propylene glycol may cause sensitisation and irritation in a small number of patients
- suitable for use at all stages of wound healing from debridement of necrotic tissue to formation of granulation tissue
- should be changed at least every one to three days
- in contact with a wound, the gel absorbs excess exudate and produces a moist environment over the surface of the wound
- can be used to soften and hydrate eschar by facilitating rehydration of the wound
- may be used where aerobic and anaerobic infection is present. For clinically infected wounds, the patient must be receiving systemic antibiotics and daily dressing changes
- use of the incorrect depth may cause some slight drying out of the gel at the edges

- the gel can be removed from the wound by irrigating with sterile sodium chloride 0.9% w/v; there may be some difficulty in doing this
- secondary dressings are required, e.g. low-adherent dressings, absorbent pads or vapour-permeable films
- N.B. product-drug interaction with povidone-iodine or iodine preparations
- in a randomised trial comparing Sterigel with Intrasite in the debridement of necrotic pressure sores, there were no significant differences in comfort, wound odour, surrounding skin condition or time to debridement[123]
- Intrasite Gel is more effective at promoting debridement than Debrisan Paste[69]
- Intrasite Gel and Debrisan Paste are both efficacious in the debridement of non-viable tissue. Intrasite Gel had a greater impact in reducing wound area; was superior in ease of application and removal, in reducing pain on application and removal; and in patient comfort during wear[70]
- Intrasite has enhanced fluid-absorbing properties but this has been achieved at the expense of the fluid-donating properties[124]
- sterile gel available pre-mixed in a unique applipak dispenser: 8g, 15g and 25g

IOBAN 2 (3M)
see VAPOUR-PERMEABLE FILMS
- polymeric film coated with a hypoallergenic adhesive on one side in which an iodophor complex is incorporated
- specifically designed as a surgical, adhesive incise drape
- provides a sustained release of iodine to the skin surface throughout use
- not recommended for use in patients with known sensitivity to iodine

IODINE
see IODOFLEX, IODOSORB
- effective against Gram-positive and Gram-negative organisms, anaerobes, fungi and yeasts, protozoa and viruses (disrupts cell proteins and lipid membranes)
- different iodine formulations are available:
  - iodine
  - cadexomer iodine
  - povidone iodine
- iodine dressings can become adherent if left to dry out on the wound
- application to large wounds or severe burns may produce systemic adverse effects such as metabolic acidosis, hypernatraemia and impairment of renal function

- *CONTRAINDICATIONS, WARNINGS.* Caution in thyroid disorders, in those receiving lithium, in pregnancy and breast feeding and use in children. May interfere with thyroid function tests
- many of the concerns about iodine are based on the toxicity of older formulations containing elemental iodine, or arise from *in vitro* studies which may not be relevant to *in vivo* situations. Newer preparations (cadexomer iodine, povidone iodine) appear to be safe, have useful antimicrobial properties and may be effective for the debridement and treatment of a variety of wounds (report of a consensus meeting,[125])

IODOFLEX (S & N, P)
see IODINE, IODOSORB POWDER and OINTMENT
- units of sterile cadexomer iodine paste containing iodine (0.9% w/w) in an inert base. The units consist of the paste sandwiched in protective gauze
- units should be changed 2–3 times per week or when there is a loss of colour
- maximum single application is 50g; weekly maximum must not exceed 150g; treatment duration should not exceed three months
- used for the topical treatment of all types of chronic wounds
- *CONTRAINDICATIONS, WARNINGS – see* IODINE. The warning relating to the co-administration of Iodoflex and sulfafurazoles and sulphonylureas has now been removed
- available in 5g, 10g and a new 17g unit which can absorb 60ml exudate

IODOSORB POWDER (S & N, P)
see IODINE and IODOSORB OINTMENT
- consists of hydrophilic beads of cadexomer impregnated with elemental iodine (0.9% w/w); cadexomer is a modified starch hydrogel
- the cadexomer absorbs exudate and forms a gel providing a moist protected environment which is conducive to wound healing. The iodine acts as an anti-infective against existing infection and prevents re-infection
- used to treat infected, medium to heavily exuding wounds
- dressings should be changed daily, or when all the beads have become saturated with wound exudate
- when the iodine has been used up, the colour changes from dark brown to white
- some patients have experienced a drawing sensation in the first hour of application
- cadexomer iodine must not be used in patients with known or suspected iodine sensitivity or thyroid disease

- if dressing dries out, saline or sterile water will wash the bulk of the dressing away. Because Iodosorb is biodegradable, any remaining Iodosorb can be left in the wound, therefore not requiring disturbance of newly-formed fragile tissue
- mild erythema without sensitisation has been reported
- *CONTRAINDICATIONS, WARNINGS* – *see* IODINE
- cadexomer iodine and dextranomer have been compared in the treatment of venous leg ulcers[126]

IODOSORB OINTMENT (S & N, P)
see IODINE and IODOSORB POWDER

- similar product to Iodosorb Powder, except in an easier-to-use formulation with an ointment base of polyethylene glycol
- used to treat chronic, light to medium exuding leg ulcers
- the ointment is less likely to cause a drawing sensation than Iodosorb Powder, because the absorption is more gradual
- the dressing should be changed approximately three times per week or when the ointment has become saturated with exudate – indicated by a loss of colour
- *CONTRAINDICATIONS, WARNINGS* – *see* IODINE
- available in 10g or 20g tubes for single use. Each 20g tube of ointment will absorb 60ml wound exudate

IRRICLENS (ConvaTec, DT)
see SODIUM CHLORIDE

- 0.9% w/v sodium chloride in a 240ml non-metered aerosol can (ozone friendly – the propellant is nitrogen)
- aerosol allows fingertip control of pressure and volume of saline; minimising wastage
- indicated for topical irrigation and cleansing of wounds; available on prescription
- each can should yield 12–15 uses of 15–20ml of saline

IV3000 (S & N, DT)
see OPSITE and VAPOUR-PERMEABLE FILMS

- consists of reactic hydrophilic polyurethane film coated with a water-based hypo-allergenic acrylic adhesive
- has a very high moisture vapour permeability which is 3 to 8 times more permeable to water vapour than conventional films
- specifically designed for intravenous catheter care

JELONET (S & N, DT)
see PARAFFIN GAUZE/TULLE GRAS
- an open-mesh leno gauze impregnated with white soft paraffin; a "normal loading" product containing 175–220g/m^2
- available packed in tins or individually wrapped

KALTOSTAT (Convatec, DT)
see ALGINATE DRESSINGS
- a sterile, absorbent dressing of non-woven calcium (80%) and sodium (20%) alginate fibre available as a wound dressing or cavity dressing
- the calcium-sodium alginate combination affords quicker gelling than calcium alginate and needs less exudate or blood to trigger the gelling action. A strong viscous gel is produced
- manufactured from a selected species of brown seaweed (*Laminaria hyperborea*) that contains guluronic acid and mannuronic acid in the proportions of 2:1
- used in the management of bleeding and non-bleeding, heavily to medium exuding wounds
- ideal for bleeding wounds
- cut or fold dressing to shape of wound
- in a clinical comparison of Kaltostat Cavity Dressing and Sorbsan Packing and Ribbon, there was no significant clinical difference in analgesic requirements, mean pain scores or bacterial counts at each dressing change. Nursing staff favoured the handling properties of Sorbsan and its availability in two product sizes[127]
- in pilonidal sinus excision wounds, both Allevyn and Kaltostat were found to be easy to use, effective and acceptable to patients and clinicians[18]
- in a randomised trial comparing Aquacel with Kaltostat, the data suggest that Aquacel may have a significantly longer wear time and reduced frequency of dressing change in patients with exuding leg ulcers[32]
- **KALTOSTAT CAVITY DRESSING** (2g): available in the DT as a soft alginate rope for cavity wounds

KERRABOOT (Ark Therapeutics Ltd, DT)
- a unique boot-shaped dressing device
- used in the management of foot and leg ulcers and other wounds of the lower leg and foot
- foot is placed in the Kerraboot and the sides pulled up and fastened with a velcro strap just below the knee; if the rectangles on the velcro straps become squares, the strap is too tight

- boot generates and maintains a warm, moist environment to optimise the healing process
- boot is a non contact dressing which encourages free drainage of exudate from the ulcer into a highly absorbent pad at the base of the boot
- boot also provides an effective barrier against wound odour
- has the potential to reduce the patient's dependency on nurses to dress and redress the ulcer
- available in small and large sizes

KETANSERIN

- serotonin (5HT) blocking drug
- encouraging results have been reported in European trials of topical ketanserin ointment in healing of leg ulcers
- workers have suggested a dual action: stimulation of granulation and collagen production in the first few days and inhibition of myofibroblast contraction (so reducing the formation of hypertrophic scars)
- not yet licensed for topical use but the oral drug is on the market as an antihypertensive agent (Serepres) in Italy

K–FOUR (Parema, DT)
see COMPRESSION BANDAGES (FOUR-LAYER)

KIKUHIME (Advancis Medical)

- a portable sub-bandage pressure monitoring kit consisting of:
  - monitor
  - 2 sensors (small and large)
  - calibration tools (screwdriver and syringe)
  - carry case
  - easy-glide (for removing a sensor from beneath a bandage)
- can be used for routine pressure monitoring, training, evaluation of technique, audit and research
- up to 3 sensors at a time can be attached to the monitor using a 3-way valve accessory

KNIT-BAND (Wilkinson Healthcare, DT)

- polyamide and cellulose contour bandage similar to K-Band and Knit Fix
- for dressing retention
- length 4-metre stretched

KNIT FIX (Robert Bailey, DT)
see BANDAGES EXTENSIBLE
- polyamide and cellulose contour bandage, Knitted BP 1988 similar to K-Band
- for dressing retention
- four sizes available

K–PLUS (Parema, DT)
see BANDAGES (EXTENSIBLE)
- a light compression bandage (type 3a)
- for the treatment of venous leg ulcers, alone or as part of a multi-layer system. It may also be used for the application of light pressure for the reduction of oedema
- applied as a spiral or as a figure of eight. Offers controlled compression of approximately 18–20mmHg at the ankle and 12–15mmHg at the calf
- available in six sizes (two of them on DT)

K–SOFT (Parema, DT)
- sub-compression wadding bandage
- used to redistribute pressure over bony prominences

K-Y LUBRICATING JELLY (J & J, DT)
- sterile water soluble medical lubricant based on polyhydric alchohols and cellulose ether
- preservatives are hydroxybenzoates (tubes) and chlorhexidine gluconate (sachets)
- contra-indicated in patients with known sensitivity to the preservatives or propylene glycol
- in a randomised, double-blind, controlled trial, a comparison was made of the relative efficacy of using Varidase in KY Jelly or KY Jelly alone. The results suggest that KY Jelly may be a cost-effective alternative to the use of Varidase in KY Jelly[128]

LARVE (Biosurgical Research Unit, SMTL Bridgend)[129]
see BIOBAG and MAGGOTS
- sterile larvae (maggots) of the common greenbottle *Lucilia sericata* (the world's "smallest surgeons")
- used to treat most types of sloughy, infected or necrotic wounds; also as an adjunct to surgery and to prepare wound sites for grafting

- maggots secrete a powerful mixture of proteolytic enzymes that breakdown slough and necrotic tissue into a semi-liquid form that can be ingested
- maggots also reduce or eliminate odour and combat infection by ingesting and killing bacteria – including MRSA[130, 131]
- may also reduce wound pain and stimulate the formation of granulation tissue
- the Prescription Pricing Authority has confirmed that prescriptions for LarvE issued by registered GPs (but not nurse prescribers) on form FP10 will be reimbursed in the normal way. Maggots are not included in the Drug Tariff as they are not medical devices – they are unlicensed medical products
- on receipt of a prescription, the pharmacist rings the order through to the Biosurgical Research Unit; the maggots are despatched by courier to arrive before noon the following day (deliveries can be made Tuesday to Saturday)
- maggots should be stored in a cool place and used on the day of receipt
- usually supplied in sterile pots, each containing about 300 maggots, priced £80 (February 2004), closed with a cap bearing a membrane filter to allow the passage of air
- applied using a dressing system that retains the maggots within the wound, allows drainage of exudate and an adequate supply of oxygen to avoid suffocation[132, 133] (for further details see the data card)
- "free range" maggots are retained within the wound with a piece of fine nylon mesh; for larger wounds, sleeve and boot nets are supplied with the maggots
- 1–5 containers are applied dependent on the size and condition of the wound; the majority of wounds treated require a maximum of 2 pots
- a simple calculator (available on request from SMTL) provides guidance on the number of pots required for a particular wound
- the quality of the maggots is assured by process validation at each stage of the production process
- maggots must be disposed of as clinical waste (a disposal container is supplied with the maggots)
- even though the use of maggots in "tea bags" is an attractive concept (to prevent the use of "free-range" maggots), it is not recommended for routine use because treatment times are greatly extended[134]
- when first applied to a wound they are only 2–3mm long but may increase in size rapidly to 8–10mm when fully grown
- generally left on a wound for a maximum of 3 days; a few treatment cycles may be required

- should not be used in wounds that have a tendency to bleed easily, or be introduced into wounds that communicate with body cavities or any internal organs. Also, should not be applied close to any large blood vessels. Maggots are of limited value in wounds covered with hard black eschar
- in the first randomised controlled comparison, there was a significant improvement in the time required to debride varicose ulcers using larvae as compared to Intrasite[135]
- granted the Millennium Product Marque
- the Biosurgical Research Unit has launched a new website for its sterile maggot business giving access to a wide range of support information: www.larve.com/
- Contact details: Biosurgical Research Unit (SMTL), Princess of Wales Hospital, Coity Road, Bridgend CF31 1RQ (Tel: 01656 752820)

LBF NO STING BARRIER FILM (CliniMed, DT)
see BARRIER FILMS
- formulated using advanced silicone technology without alcohol
- available as wipes impregnated with siloxane copolymer fluid
- applied by wiping the skin; dries in seconds with no odour when dry
- used as a peristomal skin protector for colostomies, ileostomies and urostomies
- protects against excoriating enzymes in body wastes and reduces the trauma of adhesive removal
- will not sting when applied to healthy, red, sore or excoriated skin
- free careline: 0800 585125

LEECHES (Ricarimpex SAA)
- medicinal leeches (Hirudo medicinalis) are bloodsucking aquatic animals that live in fresh water
- used as an alternative treatment to blood-letting and amputation for several thousand years reaching their height of medicinal use in the mid-1800's
- the Food and Drug Administration (FDA) has approved the commercial marketing of leeches for medicinal reasons
- can help heal skin grafts by removing blood pooled under the graft and restore blood circulation in blocked veins by removing pooled blood
- they are handled in a certified facility that tracks each lot
- the French company are the first to request and receive FDA clearance to market leeches as medical devices
- (under the Food Drug and Cosmetic Act in the USA, a medical device is an article intended to diagnose, cure, treat, prevent, or mitigate a disease or condition, or to affect a function or structure of the body, that does not achieve its primary effect through a chemical action, and is not metabolised)

LIQUIBAND – TISSUE ADHESIVE (Medlogic Global Ltd, DT)
see ADHESIVES (TISSUE), DERMABOND, EPIGLU, INDERMIL
- sterile tissue adhesive product containing 99.8% n-butyl-cyanoacrylate
- used for low tension wounds on scalp, face, trunk and limbs (wounds under tension need to have appropriate subcutaneous sutures placed prior to adhesive application)
- applied along the length of the wound either in small spots or in a continuous line – avoid adhesive entering the wound; large wounds are closed in sections
- special care is required to ensure that the wound edges are easily aligned so that no adhesive gets between the wound edges; after application, wound edges are held together for at least 30 seconds
- once in contact with the wound, the residual moisture and the natural acids within the skin promote the polymerisation process of the adhesive, resulting in a mechanical bond
- compatible with and will not cause irritation to human tissue
- do not use on hands or over joints as repetitive movement or washing will cause the adhesive to peel off
- do not apply to internal organs, blood vessels, nerve tissue or mucous membranes
- do not apply to infected or chronic wounds
- do not use on flexor or extensor surfaces
- used applicators are disposed to sharps or clinical waste
- **LIQUIBAND TISSUE ADHESIVE:** available as single use, sterile poly-propylene applicator containing 0.5g of adhesive (normal fine gauge applicator)
- **LIQUIBAND FLOW CONTROL:** as above but with a flow control safety applicator
- **LIQUIBAND SURGICAL:** combination of tissue adhesive and topical liquid barrier film dressing
- Indermil, Liquiband and Dermabond adhesives have been compared in terms of ease of use, minimal pain on application, adequate bonding time and wound closure. All produced satisfactory results in terms of wound closure and ease of use. However, Liquiband produced the most consistent results, scoring higher in most of the categories[136]

LYOFOAM (Medlock Medical, DT)
see FOAM DRESSINGS
- a neutral, polyurethane foam :
  - heat treatment of the wound contact surface renders it hydrophilic, absorbent and smooth

- the rest of the foam is hydrophobic and non-absorbent
- the smooth, shiny side is placed directly onto the wound surface
- used for open, exuding wounds of light to medium exudate
- can be left on a moist wound for up to seven days depending on exudate production
- should not be left *in situ* for extended periods in dry, shallow wounds where drying exudate may produce adhesion between the dressing and the wound
- exudate is absorbed horizontally across the hydrophilic surface; once saturated, it will become visible along the edge of the dressing (lateral strike-through)
- since the untreated foam is hydrophobic, the exudate does not pass to the outer surface of the dressing

LYOFOAM C (Medlock Medical, DT)
see DEODORISING DRESSINGS, FOAM DRESSINGS, LYOFOAM
- contains a layer of material impregnated with activated carbon between a standard Lyofoam dressing and a thin layer of polyurethane foam
- used for light to medium exuding wounds, especially those that are malodorous or infected
- exudate is absorbed horizontally across the hydrophilic surface; since the carbon layer is separated from the exudate by the hydrophobic layer, it remains dry and active throughout the life of the dressing
- no claim is made for the carbon to adsorb bacteria – because of the structure of the dressing, this is not possible
- can be used alone with the carbon (dark) side uppermost and the smooth shiny side in contact with the wound
- the use of secondary dressings will impair the effectiveness
- the $10 \times 25cm$ activated charcoal dressing will be deleted from the Drug Tariff in September 2004

LYOFOAM EXTRA (Medlock Medical, DT)
see FOAM DRESSINGS, LYOFOAM
- extra absorbent – particularly for heavily exuding wounds
- applied with the pink side facing upwards
- **Lyofoam Extra Adhesive:** also available as a dressing

LYOFOAM T (Medlock Medical)
see FOAM DRESSINGS, LYOFOAM
- polyurethane foam tracheostomy and cannula dressing ($9 \times 6.5cm$)
- made from Lyofoam with a special "cross cut" designed to fit closely around the tubes, cannulae or pins used in invasive medical procedures

LYOSHEET (Medlock Medical)
see FOAM DRESSINGS, LYOFOAM
- polyurethane foam sheet
- used as a replacement for conventional sheets to absorb exudate from severe burns
- also provides a soft padding for the patient to lie upon
- available in three, large sizes

M AND M TULLE (Malam)
see COD LIVER OIL and HONEY TULLE

MAGGOTS[137]
see BIOBAG, LarvE
- infestation by maggots (or larvae) of the order Diptera is termed myiasis[138]
- maggots are classified as unlicensed medical products
- invasion of tissues by maggots is commonly seen in tropical countries
- produce powerful proteolytic enzymes that breakdown sloughy and necrotic tissue which are ingested as a source of nutrient
- if left in the wound, maggots are effective in debriding the wound
- traditionally removed from infested wounds by using ether, chloroform, hydrogen peroxide or raw steak!
- maggots can increase wound pain, particularly in ischaemic leg ulcers. This problem is overcome by increasing the patient's analgesia, removing the maggots from the wound after 2 days instead of 3 or by using a reduced number of maggots[134]
- The Wound Care Society has published an educational leaflet on the use of sterile maggots[139]
- larvae may not survive well in wounds containing residues of some hydrogel dressings[140]
- researchers at Exeter University have set up a company to try to develop a drug that will be as effective as maggot or larvae therapy. They are focusing on the secretions from sheep blowflies. The secretions are collected, freeze-dried and turned into a powder which can be more easily applied to a wound than maggots (BBC News, 1/12/03).

MEDIPORE+PADS (3M, DT)
see NON/LOW ADHERENT DRESSINGS (similar to Cosmopor E, Mepore. Primapore, Sterifix)
- absorbent perforated dressing with adhesive border
- six sizes available

MEDI-PREP (Medlock Medical)
see ANTISEPTICS
- used for general skin preparation; cleaning cuts, wounds and abrasions; hand disinfection
- single use sachets of 1% Cetrimide BP

MEFILM (Mölnlycke, DT)
see VAPOUR-PERMEABLE FILMS
- made of polyurethane coated with a polyacrylic adhesive
- the packaging has a grid system for mapping wound size

MEFIX (Mölnlycke, DT)
- a permeable, apertured, non-woven, synthetic polyester fabric tape coated with a layer of polyacrylate adhesive
- provides secure fixation of dressings on difficult places e.g. elbows, knees, hips etc.

MELGISORB (Mölnlycke, DT)
see ALGINATE DRESSINGS
- sterile, non-woven dressing of 96% calcium and 4% sodium alginate made from brown seaweed
- used for medium to heavily exuding wounds
- available in flat and cavity sizes

MELOLIN (S & N, DT)
see NON/LOW ADHERENT DRESSINGS
- a low-adherent dressing combining a perforated polyester film wound contact layer, an absorbent 80% cotton / 20% viscose pad and a non-woven backing material
- the low-adherent plastic film side of the dressing – shiny, rough side – is placed on the wound
- performs best on light to medium exuding wounds; does not absorb excessive exudate which may cause maceration; the improved version of Melolin is 20% more absorbent
- there is some adherence to wounds because exudate may dry in the holes
- secondary dressings are needed, e.g. bandages or adhesive tapes

MELOLITE (S & N)
see NON/LOW ADHERENT DRESSINGS
- absorbent fabric pad covered on both sides by polyethylene net

MEMBRANES
see OMIDERM, SUPRASORB M, TEGAPORE.

MEPIFORM (Mölnlycke)
see SILICONE DRESSINGS
- a thin, conformable dressing consisting of a viscose nonwoven fabric bonded to a semipermeable polyurethane membrane; the inner surface of the fabric is coated with a layer of soft silicone which facilitates application and retention of the dressing to intact skin
- can be lifted from the skin without losing its adherent properties-allowing for easy re-application ('Safetac' technology)
- used to manage old and new hypertrophic and keloid scars. It may take from 3 months up to 1 year or more to improve an old scar. For prophylactic treatment, it can be used for 2–6 months depending on the condition of the scar
- dressing is worn 24 hours a day with daily inspection and washing of the skin
- a new dressing should be applied every 3–7 days or when the adherent properties of the dressing are no longer sufficient
- a waterproof dressing which can be worn during showering and bathing
- available in a range of neutral-coloured sizes which can be cut to size or shape

MEPILEX (Mölnlycke, DT)
see NON/LOW ADHERENT DRESSINGS and SILICONE DRESSINGS
- an absorbent foam pad with a vapour-permeable backing and a soft silicone layer
- designed for a wide range of exuding wounds and can be used under compression bandaging
- **Mepilex Border:** self-adherent absorbent soft silicone dressing

MEPILEX LITE (Mölnlycke, DT)
see MEPILEX
- a soft silicone wound contact dressing with a polyurethane foam film backing
- used for non to low exuding wounds e.g. diabetic foot ulcers
- should be used with care in heavily bleeding wounds
- highly conformable dressing
- can be cut to shape of wound
- can be used under compression bandaging

MEPILEX TRANSFER (Mölnlycke, DT)

see NON/LOW ADHERENT DRESSINGS and SILICONE DRESSINGS

- consists of a thin sheet of a hydrophilic open-cell polyurethane foam, coated on one surface with a layer of soft silicone, presented on a plastic film carrier
- an exudate transfer dressing - transfers exudate away from the wound
- indicated for non-exuding to heavily exuding wounds and difficult-to-treat wounds such as cancer wounds
- exudate moves vertically into a secondary absorbent pad
- use with care in heavily bleeding wounds
- thin and highly conformable which ensures direct contact to the wound and surrounding skin especially on uneven surfaces
- should be covered with a simple absorbent secondary dressing
- requires secondary fixation
- may be left undisturbed for several days on clean lightly exuding wounds
- available in large sizes which can be cut to size or shape

MEPITEL (Mölnlycke, DT)

see NON/LOW ADHERENT DRESSINGS and SILICONE DRESSINGS

- a sterile non-adhesive dressing made of a medical grade silicone gel bound to a soft and pliable polyamide net
- the netting spaces occupy 15% of the surface area and permit passage of exudate
- used for non-exuding to heavily exuding wounds (should be covered with a simple absorbent secondary dressing)
- can be left in place for up to seven days depending on the wound condition
- an aerosol spray can be used to unclog the pores of the dressing if they become blocked with slough
- in a prospective randomised trial, Mepitel reduces healing time in burned paediatric patients in comparison with silver sulfadiazine treatment[141]
- three dressings will be deleted from the October 2004 Drug Tariff: 5 × 7.5cm, 7.5 × 10cm and 10 × 18cm

MEPORE (Mölnlycke, DT)

see NON/LOW ADHERENT DRESSINGS (similar to Cosmopore E, Medipore, Primapore, Sterifix)

- apertured, non-woven polyester fabric coated with a layer of polyacrylate adhesive with an absorbent wound pad and adhesive border
- a pliable, post-operative and absorbent dressing used for many types of low to moderately exuding surgical wounds, cuts and grazes

MEPORE ULTRA (Mölnlycke, DT)
see VAPOUR-PERMEABLE FILMS
- a vapour-permeable self-adhesive film dressing with an absorbent pad
- similar to Opsite Plus and Alldress
- used for many types of low to moderately exuding superficial or postoperative wounds
- showerproof

MERCUROCHROME
see ANTISEPTICS and DYES
- mercurodibromofluorescein (an organic mercuric salt combined with fluorescein)
- usually based in alcohol which fixes skin cells and is toxic to wounds
- has the adverse effects of mercury
- dermatitis, hypersensitivity, toxicity to epidermal cells and cases of severe reactions have been reported
- only feebly active as a bacteriostatic agent
- as the hazards associated with the use of mercury compounds generally outweigh any therapeutic benefit, its clinical use should be abandoned

MESALT (Mölnlycke)
see SODIUM CHLORIDE
- an absorbent viscose/polyester non-woven dressing impregnated with sodium chloride
- indicated for the management of moderate to heavily exuding wounds in the inflammatory phase, including infected and cavity wounds
- should not be used in dry or low exuding wounds
- in contact with wound exudate, sodium chloride is released creating a hypertonic environment which absorbs the exudate together with bacteria and necrotic material from the wound
- available in three flat sizes (5 × 5cm, 7.5 × 7.5cm and 10 × 10cm) and one cavity size (2 × 100cm)

MESOFT (Mölnlycke)
- a blend of viscose and polyester fibres into a nonwoven material
- no binding agents are added ensuring that the material is extra soft
- used for cleaning wounds, absorbing fluids for pre-operative disinfeciton; can also be used as a secondary dressing
- good absorption capacity
- range of sterile and non-sterile nonwoven swabs, round sponges and split swabs available in a range of sizes

MESORB (Mesoft, Mölnlycke, DT)
see NON/LOW-ADHERENT DRESSINGS
- *see* highly absorbent cellulose dressing with a fluid-repellent backing
- used as a primary or secondary dressing for medium to heavily exuding wounds

METALLINE (Lohmann, distributed by Vernon Carus, DT)
- needle punched aluminised coating onto non-woven surface to allow fluid transmission
- the aluminium-coated side should be applied to the wound
- available as tracheostomy and drainage dressings (with pre-cut punch hole and slit)

METRONIDAZOLE
see ANABACT, ANTIBACTERIALS, METROTOP GEL[142, 143]
- actively bactericidal against anaerobic bacteria and certain protozoa; there is also some evidence for an anti-bacterial effect in certain aerobic organisms
- anaerobic organisms associated with malodour include bacteroides, *Clostridium perfringens* and *peptostreptococcus*. Aerobic organisms which produce offensive wound odours are proteus, pseudomonas and klebsiella
- controlled studies have shown a correlation between a reduction in smell and the eradication of anaerobic infection. Unfortunately continuous therapy is required because the organisms soon regrow when treatment is stopped
- can be given systemically to remove odour (200–400mg eight hourly). However metronidazole can cause nausea and long-term use is associated with neuropathy. Also the patient cannot drink alcohol during treatment
- there is a possibility that metronidazole may be absorbed after topical application; topical treatment, however, avoids many of the unwanted systemic side effects
- not always well tolerated orally
- there is also a possibility that by using metronidazole topically, antibiotic resistance may be induced. Thus the use of topical metronidazole should be restricted to fungating, malodorous tumours only
- metronidazole gel has not been compared with tablets for efficacy, speed of action or patient preference[144]
- the switch from oral to topical metronidazole in the treatment of malodorous wounds seems to have occurred on the basis of few reliable data[145]
- brand prescribing is recommended for wound care to avoid confusion with acute inflammatory exacerbation of acne rosacea products which are considerably more expensive – Metrogel (Novartis), Metrosa (Linderma), Noritate (Aventis Pharma), Rozex (Galderma) and Zyomet (Goldshield)

86

METROTOP GEL (Medlock Medical, POM)
see ANTIBACTERIALS, ANABACT, METRONIDAZOLE
- clear, colourless gel containing metronidazole BP 0.8% w/v in an aqueous hypromellose base with Benzalkonium Chloride Solution BP 0.02% v/v
- use now extended for the treatment of gravitational and pressure ulcers as well as the deodorisation of fungating, malodorous tumours
- use once or twice daily as necessary. Cavities should be loosely packed with paraffin gauze smeared in the gel
- can be re-used for single patient use for up to 28 days

MICRODON (3M)
- replaced by Medipore+ Pads

MILTON (Proctor and Gamble)
see CHLORINATED SOLUTIONS
- a stabilised 1% sodium hypochlorite solution
- when diluted 1 in 4, the solution contains 0.25% w/v available chlorine with a pH of 10.5–11.2 and is stable for several months

MINIVERSOL (Aguettant, DT)
see SODIUM CHLORIDE
- sterile, single dose polyethylene pods of liquid which are free standing
- directable jets of liquid used to rinse wounds, eyes, minor surgery
- **MINIVERSOL SODIUM CHLORIDE** – 0.9%
- **MINIVERSOL WATER**

MOLSIDOMINE
- diabetes is characterised by a nitric oxide deficiency at the wound site. Exogenous nitric oxide supplementation with the nitric oxide donor molsidomine can partially reverse impaired healing associated with diabetes by enhancing collagen synthesis and wound breaking strength[146]

MOTHER MATES (Tyco Healthcare)
see HYDROGELS
- a sterile polyurethane-based hydrophilic hydrogel disc dressing
- used for treating nipple trauma associated with breastfeeding
- protect against bacterial contamination, wound dehydration, absorb drainage and provide a cool pain-relieving cover
- dressing must be taken off prior to breastfeeding to prevent accidental choking
- available in one size at pharmacies over-the-counter

MUPIROCIN
see BACTROBAN

N-A. DRESSING (J & J, DT)
see NON/LOW ADHERENT DRESSINGS
- sterile, knitted, viscose primary dressing
- no loose fibres
- knitted open structure allows free passage of exudate through to secondary dressings
- has been improved by reducing the number of threads – dressing is now softer and more conformable

N-A ULTRA (J & J, DT)
see NON/LOW ADHERENT DRESSINGS and SILICONE DRESSINGS
(formerly called Silicone N–A)
- sterile silicone-coated knitted viscose dressing
- silicone coating is claimed to produce a non-adherent (rather than low-adherent) dressing
- silicone coating does not occlude the pores of the knitted fabric, thereby allowing drainage of exudate
- secondary dressings can be changed independently leaving N–A Ultra in position for up to 7 days

NEOSAFE – SELF ADHESIVE BORDER (Neomedic, DT)
see NON/LOW-ADHERENT DRESSINGS
- absorbent, perforated dressing with adhesive border
- similar to Cosmopor E, Medipore +, Mepore, Primapore, Sterifix and Telfa Island
- used for low to moderate exuding wounds

NEOSPORT (Neomedic, DT)
- Cotton, Polyamide and Elastane Bandage
- all bandages are not less than 4.5m in length when fully stretched
- used for support or compression

NEOTULLE (Neomedic, DT)
see PARAFFIN GAUZE/TULLE GRAS
- paraffin gauze dressing (Tulle Gras)
- normal loading – 175-220g/m^2 (similar to Jelonet)
- used for burns and chronic wounds

NEXAGON (University College London)

- a patented bio-active gel developed by UCL scientists in the Department of Anatomy and Developmental Biology
- works through manipulation of a novel target in wound healing; the gap junction (a small channel that allows cells to talk directly to their neighbours); accelerates wound healing by speeding up the rate of wound closure, reducing the degree of inflammation and reducing scar formation
- in a variety of experimental models, wounds typically close twice as fast as they would do normally e.g. an everyday cut, which would normally heal in about 7 days closes in 3 days

NIKO FIX IV (Unomedical, DT)

see VAPOUR-PERMEABLE FILMS
- for fixation of IV cannulas
- can be used for up to 3 days
- available as ported and non-ported peripheral film dressings

NON/LOW-ADHERENT DRESSINGS

see CUTILIN, INTERPOSE, MELOLIN, RELEASE, SKINTACT, SOLVALINE N, TELFA (absorbent, perforated plastic film-faced dressings)
see COSMOPOR E, MEDIPORE+PADS, MEPORE, NEOSAFE, PRIMAPORE, STERIFIX, TELFA ISLAND (absorbent, perforated dressing with adhesive border)
see N-A, N-A ULTRA, PARATEX, PRIMARY, SETOPRIME, TRICOTEX (knitted viscose primary dressing)
see MEPILEX, MEPITEL (soft silicone wound contact dressings)
see ALLDRESS, MEPORE ULTRA, OPSITE PLUS (vapour-permeable adhesive film dressings)
see EXU-DRY, MESORB (absorbent, perforated plastic film faced dressings)
see also CURITY, DRISORB, ETE, MELOLITE, PROFORE
- most are low-adherent, rather than non-adherent
- can be used on their own on dry wounds or lightly exuding wounds. A secondary dressing is required when used to dress more heavily exuding wounds
- needs to be secured with bandages or adhesive tapes

NORMASOL (Medlock Medical, DT)

see SODIUM CHLORIDE
- 25ml and 100ml sterile sachets, containing 0.9% w/v sodium chloride solution
- sachets are not as user friendly as steripods

NORMLGEL (Mölnlycke)
see HYDROGELS
- 0.9% sodium chloride gel
- used to hydrate dry wounds and to debride sloughy and necrotic wounds
- not available in the UK

NOVOGEL (Ford Medical Associates, DT)
see HYDROGELS
- a glycerine based hydrogel sheet
- consists of 65% glycerine, 17.5% polyacrylamide, 17.5% water with an outer covering of a breathable fabric
- used for dry "sloughy" or necrotic wounds; lightly exuding wounds; granulating wounds
- not suitable for infected or heavily exuding wounds
- care is needed to choose the appropriate secondary dressing
- will absorb 3–4 times its own weight
- available in squares, rectangles and circulars which can be cut to size
- **Elastogel:** similar product available in the USA

NOXYFLEX S (Geistlich Pharma, P)
- 1–2.5% solutions of noxythiolin in saline or water are sometimes used on infected wounds and burns
- potent antibacterial and antifungal activity
- exerts its effects via provision of a methylol radical
- acquired resistance does not occur and patient sensitisation is avoided
- mild discomfort on application may be relieved by addition of 2% lignocaine
- incompatible with iodine derivatives and hypochlorites

NU-GEL (J & J, DT)
see ALGINATES and HYDROGELS
- 97% hydrogel with 3% sodium alginate
- indicated for sloughy and necrotic wounds and for moist wound healing
- maintains its consistency for up to three days on the wound
- available in a 15g concertina pack

OAKMED OPTION WOUND MANAGER (Oakmed, DT)
see WOUND DRAINAGE POUCHES
- a wound drainage pouch similar to ConvaTec Wound Manager and Biotrol Draina S Fistula
- suitable for wounds with a low volume of exudate

- small, medium and large pouches are available in cut-to-fit sizes
- small, medium, large and square pouches are also available with and without access ports

OASIS (Cook)
see COLLAGEN and SKIN SUBSTITUTES
- a sterile, biomaterial derived from porcine small intestinal submucosa
- material is acellular and consists of a natural matrix of collagens and other tissue components important to the maintenance of healthy tissue
- used for the management of partial and full-thickness skin loss injuries
- the dry material is cut slightly larger than the wound, applied to the wound and then rehydrated with sterile saline (it can be rehydrated before application to the wound)
- this is then covered with a secondary dressing to maintain a moist environment – Oasis is not allowed to dry out
- during use, the dressing becomes transparent and incorporated into the granulating bed
- the wound is checked frequently and more Oasis applied if necessary at 5-10 day intervals until the wound has completely epithelialised
- when the secondary dressing is changed, a caramel-coloured gel may be observed – this should be rinsed away
- contraindicated in patients with known sensitivity to porcine material
- dressing sheets are fenestrated and available in 7, 10 and 20cm lengths

OMIDERM (distributed by Iatro Medical Systems)
see MEMBRANES
- a non-adhesive dressing of polyurethane, bonded with hydrophilic monomers; relatively inelastic when dry but upon absorption of water it becomes elastic and conforming
- can be used for superficial and partial thickness burns, abrasions and on donor sites after haemostasis has been achieved. It can also be used in a number of other granulating wounds
- not recommended for use on infected, bleeding or heavily exuding wounds; on full thickness wounds, it is only recommended as a temporary dressing
- allows up to 5L fluid transport/square metre/24 hours
- as normal healing proceeds, Omiderm peels off the healed area and should be carefully trimmed to provide a 1cm border around the wound margin. If left undisturbed it will separate spontaneously from a healed wound once epithelial cover is achieved
- membrane shrinkage and wrinkling may be a problem

- the wound site protected with Omiderm should not be immersed or heavily wetted as this may cause removal of the dressing
- dressing changes are generally not necessary unless the wound shows signs of infection, fluid accumulation, haematoma or until final peel-off. Dressing life may be up to 20 days
- the dressing is removed by wetting with sterile saline or water
- antibacterials applied to the external surface will penetrate the membrane to reach underlying tissue. However, the integrity of the membrane is lost after three days on application of silver sulphadiazine[147]
- should not be used on patients with known sensitivity to polyurethane
- available in meshed and unmeshed varieties

OMNIFIX ELASTIC (Hartmann, DT)
- elastic, permeable, apertured, non-woven, synthetic adhesive tape similar to Hypafix and Mefix
- used for wound dressing retention and for securing other medical devices e.g. catheters, cannulas

OPRAFLEX (Lohmann, distributed by Vernon Carus)
see VAPOUR-PERMEABLE FILMS
- specially designed backing material acts as an application aid and ensures accurate, wrinkle-free placement

OPRASKIN (Lohmann)
see COLLAGEN
- a sterile collagen sponge: 1cm^2 and 0.8cm thick contains 7.3mg collagen (from young calf skins) and 0.42mg (maximum) hydrogen peroxide
- used for wounds with extensive tissue damage; sponge is cut to the size and shape of the wound (and moistened before application to dry wounds)
- dressings on infected wounds are changed daily; on heavily exuding wounds – daily or several times a day; on other wounds – the dressing can be left until healed and soaked off
- contra-indicated in heavily suppurating wound cavities
- interacts with chlorine-releasing antiseptics, with albumin-precipitating substances (silver nitrate) and with caustics (iodine tincture) which denature proteins
- sponges are available in various sizes (but not in the UK)

OPSITE FLEXIGRID (S & N, DT)
see VAPOUR-PERMEABLE FILMS
- consists of a film supported on a removable flexible carrier

- film is a thin, polyurethane layer coated with a hypo-allergenic acrylic adhesive
- flexible carrier incorporates a grid system for mapping wound size (including surface area)
- can be left in place for up to 14 days

OPSITE I.V. 3000
see IV3000 film dressing

OPSITE PLUS (S & N, DT)
see VAPOUR-PERMEABLE FILMS and OPSITE
- a vapour-permeable, adhesive film formerly known as OpSite Post-Op
- similar to Alldress and Mepore Ultra
- Opsite film combined with a low-adherent, absorbent pad
- a waterproof bacteria-proof adhesive island dressing
- used for low to medium exuding wounds

OPSITE POST-OP (S & N, DT)
see OPSITE PLUS

OPSITE SPRAY DRESSING (S & N)
see BARRIER FILMS
- an acrylic copolymer, acetone/ethyl acetate spray containing no CFC propellants
- spray forms a transparent and quick-drying film which is permeable to moisture vapour and air; film can be peeled off when completely dry, left to slough off unaided or removed with adhesive plaster remover
- used for a variety of minor wounds, e.g. minor cuts, abrasions and sutures
- available over the counter

OXERUTINS (Paroven, Novartis)[148]
- licensed for "relief of symptoms of oedema associated with chronic venous insufficiency"
- evidence for the efficacy of Paroven remains unconvincing, except in lymphoedema
- for those with severe symptoms of oedema, who do not tolerate, or who get insufficient relief from support stockings, Paroven may be worth trying for four weeks, but it should be continued only if it has clearly helped
- in lymphoedema, full doses definitely seem worth trying for six months

OXYCEL (Associated Hospital Supply)
see HAEMOSTATICS
- sterile oxidised cellulose

OXYGEN
- has been used to facilitate wound healing
- good results were obtained with arterial leg ulcers when periods of hyperbaric oxygen were interspersed with periods of tissue hypoxia when oxygen therapy was withheld[149]
- supplemental oxygen given during and after colorectal resection reduces the incidence of surgical wound infection by half[150]
- hyperbaric oxygen can be used as an adjunctive therapy to promote healing in problematic wounds[151]
- there is some evidence that people with diabetic foot ulcers are less likely to have a major amputation if they receive hyperbaric oxygen therapy. This is based on 3 randomised trials with a limited number of patients. Further research is required[152]
- a recent Cochrane review concluded that the routine management of chronic ulcers of the lower limb (diabetic foot ulcers, venous and arterial ulcers and pressure ulcers) with hyperbaric oxygen therapy is not justified by the existing evidence[152]

PARAFFIN GAUZE/TULLE GRAS (non-medicated)
see JELONET, NEOTULLE, PARANET, PERITEX, UNITULLE
- bleached cotton/rayon cloth impregnated with white or yellow soft paraffin (tulle gras equivalent to "greased net")
- dressings contain different weights of paraffin per unit area e.g.
  - Jelonet (normal loading, 175–220g/m^2)
  - Paranet 10 × 10cm (light loading, 90–130g/m^2)
  - Paranet in tins (normal loading)
  - Unitulle (light loading)
- paraffin reduces the adherence of the dressing to the wound if applied in sufficient thickness
- used as a primary wound dressing for clean, superficial wounds, e.g. abrasions, cuts or partial thickness burns; heavier loaded paraffins are used for skin graft transfer
- antibacterials can be dispersed in the soft paraffin but water-soluble medicaments may not be readily released into the wound; this results in variable efficacy
- requires secondary dressings, e.g. absorbent pads

- said to be semi-permeable and non-adherent but there may be some adherence due to the sticky nature of the paraffin which is difficult to remove from the wound with aqueous wound cleansing agents
- needs frequent changing to avoid drying out and incorporation in granulation tissue

PARANET (Vernon-Carus, DT)
see PARAFFIN GAUZE/TULLE GRAS
- 10 × 10cm dressing is light loaded with yellow soft paraffin, 90–130g/m², (sachets)
- dressings in tins are normal loaded with yellow soft paraffin

PARATEX (Parema, DT)
see NON/LOW ADHERENT DRESSINGS
- a non/low-adherent dressing similar to N-A, N-A Ultra, Setoprime, Tricotex
- a knitted viscous primary dressing
- the 12.5 × 14.5cm size has been deleted from the Drug Tariff (9.5 × 9.5cm is still available)

PAROVEN (Novartis)
see Oxerutins

PASTE BANDAGES
- medicated paste bandages are used in the treatment of skin conditions associated with leg ulcers, e.g. eczema, inflammation
- are applied from the base of the toes to the tibial tuberosity (with the foot at right angles); additional bandaging is always required
- can be left *in situ* for 1–2 weeks before a further dressing is required; act as a buffer between the fragile, inflamed skin and the turns of the compression bandage
- are able to absorb exudate
- many patients are sensitive to some of the constituents of paste bandages such as parabens preservatives, lanolin, etc. It is advisable before using paste bandages, to patch test the patient with a small strip of bandage to the leg for at least 48 hours
- paste bandages are occlusive bandages which may increase absorption of topical medicaments, e.g. steroids
- there are many types of paste bandage available (individually wrapped, 7.5cm × 6m)
- Viscopaste PB7 and Ichthopaste are in the Drug Tariff

- Steripaste, Zincaband, Icthaband, Quinaband and Calaband (Medlock Medical products) have all been deleted from the Drug Tariff but remain prescribable as a medicinal product
- Coltapaste and Tarband have been discontinued

Zinc Paste Bandages
- bandages of choice for patients who display multiple sensitivities
- protective, soothing applications for reddened, irritated skin
- **STERIPASTE** (Medlock Medical) consists of an open-wove bleached cotton bandage impregnated evenly with a paste of zinc oxide 15% w/w. Also contains glycerol, coconut oil, aluminium magnesium silicate, xanthan gum, polysorbate 80, sorbitan-mono-oleate, synthetic spermaceti and purified water. Unique preservative-free formulation. A patch test study has not shown any convincing allergic reactions. It should be used cautiously in patients allergic to cetylstearyl alcohol and avoided in those allergic to a sorbitan ester[153]
- **VISCOPASTE PB7** (S & N, DT) consists of an open-wove bleached cotton bandage impregnated evenly with a paste containing zinc oxide (10%), glycerol, cetostearyl alcohol, cetomacrogol, white oil, guar gum, xanthum gum, methyl and propyl parabens preservatives and water
- when compared to Kaltostat and a zinc oxide-impregnated stockinette, Viscopaste significantly improved the healing of chronic venous ulcers when used in combination with compression bandaging[154]
- **ZINCABAND** (Medlock Medical) consists of an open-wove bleached cotton bandage impregnated evenly with a paste of zinc oxide (15%), modified starch, glycerine, castor oil, citric acid, hydroxybenzoate and water.

Zinc paste and calamine bandage
- action is mainly emollient: soothes irritated, fragile skin surrounding ulcer, e.g. erythema, eczema and dermatitis
- **CALABAND** (Medlock Medical) consists of an open-weave bleached cotton bandage impregnated evenly with a paste of zinc oxide (9.25%), calamine, modified starch, citric acid, glycerine, castor oil, phenosept and water

Zinc paste, calamine and clioquinol bandage
- action is anti-bacterial and deodorant
- suitable for grossly infected, offensive ulcers
- **QUINABAND** (Medlock Medical) consists of an open-wove bleached cotton bandage impregnated evenly with a paste of zinc oxide (9.25%),

clioquinol (1%), calamine (5.75%), modified starch, citric acid, glycerine, castor oil, teepol, phenoxyethanol and water. Clioquinol is a broad-spectrum antibacterial agent of low sensitising potential. Use of Quinaband may result in elevation of serum protein-bound iodine levels

Zinc paste and coal tar bandage
– during normal treatment granulation will occasionally cease; short-term use of this bandage will often restart the process
– has anti-inflammatory and mild antiseptic properties
– used for dry and scaly skin, e.g. eczema, dermatitis, lichenification
– **COLTAPASTE** (S & N) and **TARBAND** (SSL) have been discontinued

Zinc paste and ichthammol bandages
– action is mainly anti-inflammatory
– may irritate or sensitise skin
– used to soothe irritated skin, e.g. eczema, when tar is not tolerated
– **ICTHABAND** (Medlock Medical) consists of an open-wove bleached cotton bandage impregnated evenly with a paste of zinc oxide (15%), ichthammol (2%), modified starch, glycerine, castor oil, citric acid, propyl hydroxybenzoate and water
– **ICHTHOPASTE** (S & N, DT) consists of an open-wove bleached cotton bandage impregnated evenly with a paste consisting of zinc oxide (6%), ichthammol (2%), glycerin, gelatin, cyclonette wax and phenoxetol

PEHA-CREPP E (Hartmann, DT)
see BANDAGES EXTENSIBLE
• synthetic conforming bandage
• used for dressing retention

PENTOXIFYLLINE (Trental, Aventis Pharma, POM)[155]
• improves the delivery of oxygen in ischaemic tissues, has fibrinolytic effects that are possibly mediated by leucocytes, and reduces the adhesion of polymorphonuclear leucocytes
• these properties might explain the clinical benefit of pentoxifylline when added to a standard regimen of dressing and compression bandaging in increasing the healing rates of resistant venous ulcers. Treatment may need to be continued for several months.
• appears to be an effective adjunct to compression bandaging for treating venous ulcers. In the absence of compression, may be effective for treating venous ulcers. The majority of adverse effects are likely to be tolerated by

patients, and gastrointestinal disturbances (indigestion, diarrhoea and nausea) are the most frequent[156]

- the difference in the healing rates of venous leg ulcers between patients taking pentoxifylline and placebo did not reach statistical significance[157]
- in a randomised control trial of 172 patients with chronic venous hypertension, 67% of patients in the pentoxifylline group had a completely healed ulcer after 6 months compared to 31% in the placebo group[158]
- in a randomised control trial of 85 patients with venous ulcers, 88% of patients in the pentoxifylline group had a completely healed ulcer after 12 months compared to 44% in the placebo group[159]
- in a systematic review[160] of nine randomised controlled trials involving a total of 572 patients, the trials compared pentoxifylline against placebo, with or without compression. The results suggest that pentoxifylline gives additional benefit to compression for venous leg ulcers, and is possibly effective for patients not receiving compression. The majority of adverse effects are gastrointestinal disturbances

PERITEX (Southon-Horton)
see PARAFFIN GAUZE/TULLE GRAS

PERMAFOAM (Hartmann, DT)
see FOAMS

- Polyurethane Foam Film dressing
- used for moderate to heavily exuding wounds
- the intense swelling of the foam matrix in a vertical direction helps to conform to wounds which are rugged
- available in square and rectangular dressings
- **PERMAFOAM** is available without an adhesive border
- **PERMAFOAM COMFORT** is available with an adhesive border

PERMITABS (Centrapharm)
see POTASSIUM PERMANGANATE

- purple, bi-convex, soluble tablets containing Potassium Permanganate BP 400mg
- a quantity of the required strength of solution may be prepared by dissolving the appropriate number of tablets in warm water, e.g. 1 tablet dissolved in 4 litres of water provides a 0.01% (1 in 10,000) solution
- the tablets should be handled as little as possible to avoid staining the fingers
- avoid getting the solution into the eyes, nose or mouth

PHENOXYETHANOL
see ANTISEPTICS
- is effective against strains of *Pseudomonas aeruginosa* but is less effective against other Gram-negative and Gram-positive organisms
- may be used as a 2% aqueous solution or cream

PHENYTOIN
- has been used in the healing of pressure sores, venous stasis and diabetic ulcers, traumatic wounds and burns[161] and large abscess cavities[162]. All the studies have reported enhancement of wound healing, with insignificant adverse effects
- phenytoin reduces oedema and inflammation, separates slough and accelerates the growth of granulation tissue. Phenytoin may promote wound healing by a number of mechanisms, including stimulation of fibroblast proliferation, facilitation of collagen deposition, glucocorticoid antagonism and antibacterial activity[161]
- early administration of topical phenytoin in the treatment of stage II pressure ulcers significantly accelerates healing and prevents progression to stage III or IV wounds according to the results of a randomised trial[163]
- patients receiving topical phenytoin should be monitored for signs of systemic toxicity as measurable phenytoin plasma concentrations are obtained

PHYSIOTULLE (Coloplast, DT)
- soft polymer wound contact dressing similar to Tegapore and Urgotul
- non-occlusive, wound contact layer that resembles traditional gauze, although it is coated with a vaseline containing carboxymethylcellulose which absorbs exudate and prevents adherence (hydrocolloid based wound contact layer)
- suitable for superficial burns, donor sites, post operative wounds, skin abrasions, pressure ulcers and leg ulcers

PNEUMATIC COMPRESSION (EXTERNAL) (EPC)
- EPC is also known as intermittent pneumatic compression (IPC) therapy
- used to reduce venous stasis by compressing the superficial veins and forcing blood into the deep veins
- air is used as the compression medium
- EPC devices are sleeve- or boot-shaped chambers that fill with air and electrical pumps with gauges that provide intermittent compression to the lower extremities
- mainly used in preventing deep vein thrombosis (DVT), but it also acts as an adjuvant therapy for skin ulcers and limb oedema

- modifications have been made to IPC devices to enhance their functions by providing external pressure that simulates diastolic blood pressure
- in a pre-assessment of the literature, since 1976, 25 randomised controlled trials have been conducted to assess the clinical efficacy of EPC therapy for patients with venous insufficiency (VI); 5 systematic reviews regarding the efficacy of EPC therapy were identified
- EPC reduces the risk of deep vein thrombosis for patients who cannot walk due to trauma, joint surgery or neurosurgery. There is still limited evidence, however, supporting the effect of EPC on the healing of venous ulcers and other disorders resulting from chronic VI[164]

POLYSKIN II (Tyco Healthcare, DT)
see VAPOUR-PERMEABLE FILMS
- a vapour-permeable adhesive polyurethane film dressing with patented two-tab delivery system
- used for dry to light exuding wounds, for autolytic debriding and as a secondary dressing
- allows moisture and oxygen vapour transfer (MVTR of 585g/sqm/24hrs)
- impermeable to liquids and semi-occlusive
- **POLYSKIN MR** (DT)
- a moisture responsive, vapour-permeable adhesive dressing
- solvent-based acrylic adhesive diamond pattern (80-90%)
- allows moisture and oxygen vapour transfer (MVTR of 4800g/sqm/24hrs)

POLYVINYLCHLORIDE FILM
see VAPOUR-PERMEABLE FILMS
- plasticised, thin, clear, sheeting that was originally produced for wrapping foodstuffs (as Clingfilm, Wrapfilm, etc.)
- cheap, easy to apply, comfortable to wear, pain-free to remove and transparent
- non-sterile
- has been used in burns units for dressings before the ward round, before surgery and when the patient is transferred from casualty to the burns unit

POTASSIUM PERMANGANATE
see DYES, PERMITABS
- stains the skin brown
- daily 15 minute soaks are used as an astringent in concentrations of 1 in 8000 to 1 in 10,000 to cleanse and deodorise suppurating eczematous wounds and acute dermatoses

POVIDONE-IODINE
see ANTISEPTICS, BETADINE, INADINE, IODINE, SAVLON DRY, VIDENE
- an iodophore which is a loose complex of iodine and a carrier – povidone
- iodine is gradually released from the iodophore and has the broadest spectrum of activity of any antiseptic commonly available. In a comparative trial against 33 strains of methicillin resistant *Staph. aureus* (MRSA), chlorhexidine achieved full efficacy against only three strains of MRSA, whilst povidone-iodine was fully effective against every single strain on trial[46]
- has largely displaced the numerous antibiotic-containing ointments
- because of the slow release, povidone-iodine is less potent and less toxic than preparations containing free iodine
- in both an experimental and clinical study, povidone iodine did not cause any adverse reactions or have an adverse affect on wound healing[165]
- allergic contact dermatitis and one case of anaphylaxis have been reported[166]
- avoid use on large wounds as excessive absorption of iodine may occur
- antibacterial effect is reduced by contact with pus and exudate so the preparations must be applied at intervals sufficiently short for brown coloration to persist. Active iodine is brown; on inactivation, iodine is converted to colourless iodides
- does not cause permanent staining to skin or clothes
- alcoholic solutions should not be used
- its use has been extensively reviewed[167]. Its therapeutic benefit in open wounds has been supported in some reviews but questioned by others because of delayed wound healing and iodine toxicity
- new formulations are under test e.g. povidone-iodine liposome hydrogel

PRIMAPORE (S & N, DT)
see NON/LOW-ADHERENT DRESSINGS (similar to Cosmopore E, Medipore, Mepore, Sterifix)
- absorbent, perforated dressing with a Melolin-like low-adherent absorbent pad and an adhesive border
- indicated for post-operative use and also for cuts, lacerations and sutured wounds

PRIMARY (Robinson, DT)
see NON/LOW ADHERENT DRESSING
- knitted viscous primary dressing similar to N-A, Paratex, Setoprime and Tricotex
- available in 9.5 × 9.5cm and 12.5 × 14.5cm sizes

PRIMSKIN (Spenco Healthcare International)
see HYDROGELS
- a flat, sheet, transparent hydrogel dressing containing up to 96% water and 4% polyethylene oxide on a polyethylene mesh support to provide strength (formerly known as Spenco 2nd Skin)
- the gel is covered with one clear polyester and one blue polyethylene film; the blue film is discarded for use in the occlusive mode; both films are discarded for use in the non-occlusive mode
- used for superficial wounds e.g. suture lines, post-operative wounds, abrasions
- available in sterile and non-sterile forms; only the sterile dressing should be used for wounds

PROFLAVINE (DT)
see ANTISEPTICS
- a brightly coloured acridine derivative available as:
  - Proflavine solution – 0.1% aqueous solution of proflavine hemisulphate
  - Proflavine Cream BPC – 0.1% water in oil (w/o) emulsion containing wool fat
  - Proflavine Cream – 0.1% oil in water emulsion (o/w)
- slow-acting antiseptic; mildly bacteriostatic against many Gram-positive bacteria but less effective against Gram-negative organisms e.g. *Proteus* spp., *Pseudomonas* spp. and *Escherichia coli*
- hypersensitivity reactions have been reported occasionally (the cream contains wool fat, a known sensitising agent)
- a w/o proflavine cream has little or no antibacterial activity as the proflavine is not released from the emulsion base; o/w emulsions should overcome this problem[168]
- proflavine creams do not offer any advantages over more modern alternatives. Calcium alginate (Sorbsan) is superior to traditional gauze soaked in proflavine in acute surgical wounds and abscesses in terms of comfort of dressing and bacterial clearance[169]
- in a randomised, controlled trial to compare the cost benefits of Aquacel and Proflavine gauze in acute surgical wounds, Aquacel gave considerable savings. Aquacel facilitated earlier discharge from hospital, was less expensive per patient episode and avoided the need for anaesthesia for dressing changes[170]

PROFORE (S & N, DT)
see COMPRESSION BANDAGES (FOUR-LAYER)
- also available as a wound contact layer

PROFORE #1 (S & N, DT)
- 100% viscose fleece
- a sub-compression wadding bandage used as a component of multi-layer compression bandaging

PROGUIDE 2 LAYER SYSTEM (S & N, DT)
see COMPRESSION BANDAGES (TWO-LAYER)
- a two-layer compression bandaging kit consisting of:
  - Absorbent padding layer – applied in a spiral format from toe to knee with an ankle lock, 50% overlap and no pressure
  - Vari-stretch compression layer – applied in a spiral format at 50% extension from toe to knee with an ankle lock and 50% overlap using centre line as a guide
- the kit also contains a primary dressing to cover the wound
- used for the treatment of venous leg ulcers
- delivers optimum compression between 30–70% stretch whilst avoiding the dangers of over compression
- a coloured centre line enables correct application at 50% overlap
- the correct extension is obtained when the printed oval containing 2 intersecting lines changes to a circle with intersecting lines forming a right angle
- an evaluation study suggests that each bandage should be partially pre-stretched prior to application, particularly when bandaging limbs with a circumference towards the lower end of the recommended range[57]
- healing rates comparable to Profore (4-layer bandage)
- less bulk for patient comfort
- faster application
- maintains optimal sub-bandage pressure for up to 7 days
- does not contain the known sensitisers, latex, thiuram or colophony
- available in 3 sizes for different ankle circumferences:
  - Red – ankle circumference 18–22cm
  - Yellow – ankle circumference 22–28cm
  - Green – ankle circumference 28–32cm

PROMOGRAN (J & J, DT)
see COLLAGEN dressings
- an hexagonal collagen dressing (Drug Tariff classifies it as a Protease Modulating Matrix)
- a matrix of 55% freeze-dried collagen and 45% oxidised regenerated cellulose (ORC)

- used to treat chronic wounds that are free of necrotic tissue and visible signs of infection
- applied directly to the wound and covered by a moist healing dressing; it forms a gel and is gradually absorbed into the wound
- both collagen and ORC are completely bio-absorbable and re-treatment is easily added to the wound (residual dressing does not need to be removed):
  - re-apply every 1–2 days for heavy exudate
  - re-apply every 2–3 days for medium-low exudate
- for very dry wounds, sterile saline should be used to hydrate each sheet prior to application (to initiate the gelling process)
- improves healing by
  - actively binding and inactivating proteases that degrade endogenous growth factors and impede healing
  - binding and protecting growth factors which are released into the wound as the dressing is absorbed thereby allowing healing to progress naturally
- both collagen and ORC are haemostats (i.e. they assist in stopping bleeding by providing a matrix for the clot)
- contraindicated in patients with known hypersensitivity to ORC or collagen
- available in 2 sizes – 28 × 28cm and 123 × 123cm

PURILON GEL (Coloplast, DT)
see ALGINATES and HYDROGELS
- a hydrogel/alginate gel consisting of calcium alginate, CMC and more than 90% water
- primarily used for dry and moist necrotic wounds. Can also be used as a supplement to moist wound healing in general
- hydrates necrotic tissue and effects debridement
- absorbs debris and excess exudate
- requires a secondary dressing on top of the gel
- gel changing interval may be up to 3 days
- available in 8g and 15g sizes

REGRANEX (Janssen-Cilag, POM)
see GROWTH FACTORS
- clear, colourless to straw-coloured gel containing becaplermin 100µg/g (0.01%)
- a recombinant human platelet derived growth factor (rhPDGF–BB)
- promotes the chemotactic recruitment and proliferation of cells involved in wound repair – the predominant effect is to enhance the formation of granulation tissue

- used for full thickness, neuropathic, chronic, diabetic ulcers less than or equal to 5cm^2
- applied once daily as a continuous thin layer to the entire ulcerated area and covered by a moist saline gauze dressing (not occlusive dressings)
- therapy should be continued to a maximum of 20 weeks as long as healing progress is seen on periodic evaluations
- contra-indicated for known hypersensitivity to any ingredient e.g. parabens preservatives, or for known neoplasm at or near the site of application (as becaplermin is a growth factor)
- use within six weeks after first opening
- store in the refrigerator at 2–8°C (do not freeze)
- safety and effectiveness have not been established in children and adolescents below the age of 18 years
- side effects reported in clinical trials: infection, skin ulceration, skin disorder, including erythema and pain, bullous eruption and oedema
- the net price is £275 for a 15g tube – a course of treatment is likely to cost between £550 and £825
- may be a cost-effective treatment for neuropathic diabetic foot ulcers in a wide range of European settings. In the UK, becaplermin may even be cost saving[171]

RELEASE (J & J, DT)
see NON/LOW ADHERENT DRESSINGS
- low adherent ethylene methyl acrylate film wrapped around an absorbent core of viscose rayon sandwiched between two layers of non-woven fabric
- used for low to medium exuding wounds
- highly conformable

REPLICARE ULTRA (S & N, DT)
see HYDROCOLLOIDS
- used for light to medium exuding wounds
- available as square and anatomically shaped sacral, thin dressings

REPOSE (Frontier Therapeutics)
- The University Hospital of Wales, Cardiff has developed the **Repose** system of mattresses and cushions to prevent pressure sores
- utilises high-tech materials in a low-tech manner at low cost
- products are packed inside a pump which enables them to be easily inflated and ready for use within seconds

ROEHAMPTON BURNS DRESSING (Relyon)
- sterile first-aid foam dressing for application to burned areas, to protect against additional trauma and contamination and to provide protection in transit
- indicated for 1st, 2nd and 3rd degree burns

ROSIDAL K (Vernon-Carus, DT)
- a short stretch compression bandage similar to Actiban, Actico, Comprilan, Silkolan and Varex Short Stretch
- used for venous leg ulcers and lymphodema

SAVLON DRY POWDER (Novartis)
see ANTISEPTICS and POVIDONE-IODINE
- 1.14% povidone-iodine dry powder spray in an aerosol (for minor wounds)

SEASORB (Coloplast, DT)
see ALGINATES and HYDROCOLLOIDS
- an alginate containing hydrocolloid dressing formerly called Seasorb
- consists of 85% calcium alginate and 15% carboxymethylcellulose
- used for medium to heavily exuding wounds (good absorption capacity)
- as the gel structure is cohesive, the dressing is easily removed in one piece
- **SeaSorb Soft Dressings** - 3 sizes available
- **SeaSorb Soft Filler:** for cavity wounds

SEPRAFILM (Genzyme)
see HYALURONIC ACID
- Genzyme is developing a family of surgical products designed to reduce adhesion formation in a wide range of surgical procedures
- these products are made from hyaluronic acid, a biopolymer produced naturally by the body to lubricate and protect tissues
- **Seprafilm:** first of these products to reach the market; it is a bioresorbable membrane, a film that looks like a sheet of waxed paper. It is used to separate and protect tissues damaged by incisions, suturing or cauterisation
- **Sepracoat coating solution:** a liquid formulation of hyaluronic acid used to treat incidental damage to internal tissues as a result of handling and drying due to exposure
- **Sepragel bioresorbable gel:** an investigational product used for surfaces that are inaccessible to Seprafilm during open surgery

SETOPRIME (Medlock Medical, DT)
see NON/LOW ADHERENT DRESSINGS

SILASTIC FOAM
see CAVI-CARE (relaunched in April 1994 by S & N)

SILGEL (Nagor, DT)
see SILICONE DRESSINGS
- silicone gel (polysiloxane) products available as gel and sheets
- for the management of hypertrophic and keloid scars and associated erythema following carbon dioxide lasers, chemical peels and dermabrasion
- do not use on open or infected wound, scab or stitches
- best results are achieved during a period of 2-4 months (sometimes much longer)
- **SILGEL Gel:** consists of 100% polysiloxane in a 20ml tube; should be used sparingly and is gently massaged to affected area offering 24 hour scar management; once dry, cosmetics may be applied; gel is suitable for visible areas, on joints and crevices and for children
- the beneficial effects of silicone cream have been demonstrated on scars and keloid[172] and on grafted skin[173]
- **SILGEL Sheets:** consist of 100% polysiloxane available in a variety of anatomical shapes including abdominal, submammary and circular; softens scar tissue and contractures; sheet is washed daily with a mild soap solution and will last for several weeks in use

SILICONE DRESSINGS
see ADVASIL, CICA-CARE, MEPIFORM, MEPILEX, MEPITEL, N–A ULTRA, SILGEL, SILICONE GEL, SIL–K FILM
- silicones are polymers (long chains) of oxygen and silicone (with attached organic groups); the degree of polymerisation determines the physical form of the silicone e.g. a thin oil, hard rubber or resin
- dressings are coated with soft silicone as an adhesive or a wound contact layer and do not cause trauma on removal
- available in different forms:
  - atraumatic wound contact layers
  - absorbent dressings for exuding wounds
  - dressings for the treatment of hypertrophic scars and keloids
- evidence-based clinical recommendations support the use of silicone gel sheeting as a first line therapy on immature, linear and widespread burn hypertrophic scars and minor keloids. Silicone gel sheeting should also be considered as a first line prophylactic measure to help prevent the development of hypertrophic scars or keloids after surgery[174]
- currently it is believed that silicone gel works by promoting hydration of the scar

- silicones are chemically inert and adverse effects are rare
- a list of frequently asked questions about soft silicone dressings (Mepitel, Mepilex etc) is available at: www.worldwidewounds.com/2003/october/Thomas

SILICONE GEL SHEETS (Spenco Healthcare International)
see SILICONE DRESSINGS
- consists of chemically inert, transparent and conformable pure silicone gel
- used to reduce hypertrophic and keloid scarring
- used successfully to flatten scar tissue, increase elasticity and reduce discoloration, regardless of degree, site or age – making the scar cosmetically more acceptable
- gel sheets may be sterilised in an autoclave; the sheets are re-usable and can be washed in warm water or mild antiseptic solution.

SIL-K FILM (Degania)
see SILICONE DRESSINGS
- soft, durable and transparent silicone sheet less than 1mm thick
- indicated for keloid and hypertrophic scars
- transparent sheet allows users to see their scars improving over the two to nine month period advocated for use; can be re-used for many months

SILKOLAN (Parema, DT)
see BANDAGES EXTENSIBLE
- short stretch compression bandage (similar to Comprilan)
- two sizes available

SILVER[175]
see ACTICOAT, ACTISORB SILVER 220, AQUACEL AG, ARGLAES, AVANCE, CONTREET, FLAMAZINE, SILVER NITRATE, URGOTUL SSD
- silver metal or its salts have antiseptic and antibacterial properties
- silver metal does not readily interact with the skin but in the presence of wound exudate, silver ionises to release reactive silver ions
- possible reasons for the antibacterial effects of silver[175, 176]:
  - cytoplasmic poison in bacteria and fungi
  - denatures cytoplasmic and mitochondrial enzymes and nuclear proteins
  - interference with bacterial electron transport
  - binding to DNA of bacteria and their spores thus increasing the stability of the double helix and impairing cell replication
  - cell membrane interaction – structural and receptor function damage

- formation of insoluble, and by implication, metabolically ineffective, compounds
- present knowledge of the uptake and metabolism of silver by various cell types is imperfectly understood
- the ideal silver dressing will deliver silver in a sustained therapeutic way achieving an effective antibacterial dose with limited opportunity for systemic absorption; this is preferable to the use of silver solutions or creams
- silver dressings can be used for the treatment of infected acute and chronic wounds
- depending on the wound, dressings can be changed every 1–7 days but should not be used for more than 10 weeks
- silver compounds may react with environmental pollutants to form black silver sulphide – a general grey discoloration (argyria) which is largely a cosmetic problem[84]. Prolonged use of silver nitrate solutions are more likely to cause this than silver dressings. There are no reports of argyria caused by modern wound dressings containing silver
- the potential for silver allergy and hypersensitivity is well documented
- the antimicrobial activity of 4 silver dressings have been compared against three micro-organisms in a laboratory-based study[177]. Analysis of the silver content of each dressing indicates major differences:
  - Acticoat   109mg/100cm^2
  - Contreet-H   31.2–32.4mg/100cm^2
  - Actisorb Silver 220   2.43–2.95mg/100cm^2
  - Avance   1.59mg/100cm^2
- the authors surmised from their results that Acticoat would be likely to be the most effective dressing for killing bacteria within a wound. Contreet-H would also have an effect if left in place for an extended period, as is usual with hydrocolloid dressings. Actisorb Silver 220 and Avance would be likely to perform less well

SILVER NITRATE
see ANTISEPTICS and SILVER
- longest history of all silver compounds
- formerly used as a 10% solution combined with tannic acid
- highly caustic and astringent at concentrations above 2%
- 0.5% aqueous solution used for short periods only, then reduce to 0.25%
- use for 2–3 days only to avoid toxicity
- has a broad anti-bacterial spectrum (bacteriostatic)
- inexpensive and readily available
- sometimes used if acetic acid is ineffective against pseudomonas colonisation but has largely been replaced by Flamazine

- painless on application and does not cause local sensitivity
- major disadvantage of staining tissues brown-black, making it difficult to delineate between healing and necrotic tissue (argyria)
- may affect the patient's electrolyte and water balance
- can cause methaemoglobinaemia and metabolic disturbances
- overgranulation is sometimes treated using 0.25% compresses, or with a silver nitrate stick for more exuberant tissue, and curettage if necessary

SILVER SULFADIAZINE
see FLAMAZINE

SKIN-PREP (S & N)
see BARRIER FILMS
- contains isopropyl alcohol, butyl ester of PVM/MA copolymer, acetyl tributyl citrate
- available as wipes, aerosol and brush-on form
- protects sensitive skin when used under ostomy appliances, adhesive bandaging, orthopaedic plaster casts
- sting will be experienced if Skin-Prep contacts cut or open wounds
- can reduce erythema caused by trauma from skin tapes[178]

SKIN SUBSTITUTES[95, 179]
see AMNION, APLIGRAF, BIOBRANE, DERMAGRAFT, INTEGRA, OASIS
- some are synthetic/biosynthetic e.g. Dermagraft, Integra, OrCel, TransCyte
- some are biological e.g. Alloderm, Apligraf, Durasis, Mediskin I, Oasis, Surgisis
- some are tissue engineered products using living cells (fibroblasts, keratinocytes) together with natural or synthetic extracellular matrices as scaffolds which provide mechanical stability and a three-dimensional framework for subsequent tissue infiltration and development
- biodegradable scaffold materials are often used – these are resorbed as new tissue is laid down
- natural scaffolds are derived from human or animal tissues e.g. collagen and hyaluronan
- synthetic scaffolds can be manufactured on a large scale e.g. polyglycolic acid and polylactic acid
- cells consist of three types:
  - *Epidermal:* grafts of cultured epidermal cells with no dermal components e.g. cultured autologous epidermal cells, cultured allogenic epidermal

cells, Epicel, LaserSkin. Culture time may be prolonged and there may be difficulties with handling
- *Dermal:* helps to prevent wound contraction and provides greater mechanical stability e.g. allogenic skin, bovine collagen, Alloderm, Biobrane, Dermagraft
- *Combined Dermal/Epidermal:* e.g. composite cultured skin, Apligraf. Care must be taken to apply the dermal layer in contact with the wound bed
- used for burns and more difficult, recalcitrant wounds
- promote wound healing by stimulating the host to produce a variety of cytokines
- the condition of the wound bed will affect product efficacy
- advantages: readily available; do not require painful and invasive procedures; may be used in out-patients
- disadvantages: high cost; potential disease transmission; limited viability (do not survive indefinitely)
- a code of practice applies to organisations that supply products that use material of human origin to the health service for therapeutic purposes. In order to provide safe human-derived therapeutic products of reliable quality, good practice standards need to be observed in the selection of donors, retrieval of tissues, testing, processing, storage and delivery. This code addresses these issues and applies to wound dressings modified by the application of human-derived growth factors and to bioengineered skin substitutes and to other therapeutic products[180]

SKINTACT (Robinson, DT)
see NON/LOW ADHERENT DRESSINGS
- absorbent, perforated plastic film faced, dressing
- apertured film on both sides of dressing alleviates worry of dressing being applied incorrectly
- cotton absorbent pad of dressing can cope with low to medium exuding wounds

SMOKING AND WOUND HEALING
- smoking has long been suspected to adversely affect wound healing
- the components of cigarette smoke that are of greatest interest to poor wound healing are:
  - nicotine which causes vasoconstriction and decreased tissue perfusion;
  - carbon monoxide which causes tissue hypoxia;
  - hydrogen cyanide which inhibits enzyme systems;
- "second-hand" smoke may delay wound repair because of the inability of the fibroblasts to migrate into the wounded area leading to a build up of

connective tissue causing fibrosis and excess scarring[181]
- health professionals have a role in providing evidence-based smoking cessation interventions to improve the outcome for patients with wounds[182]

SODIUM CHLORIDE
see CURASALT, IRRICLENS, MESALT, MINIVERSOL, NORMASOL, SODIUM CHLORIDE,
- sterile solutions of 0.9% w/v sodium chloride available in aerosols, sachets and ampoules (Steripods), ideal for topical irrigation and cleansing of wounds
- safe, non-irritant and non-toxic
- has no antiseptic properties but dilutes the concentrations of bacteria in the wound
- a warmed saline solution used as a wound irrigant on anaesthetised lacerations is preferred by patients, although the warmth has no affect on pain scores[183]

SODIUM CHLORIDE STERIPODS (Medlock Medical)
see SODIUM CHLORIDE
- sterile solution of sodium chloride 0.9% w/v in purified water (20ml); Steripods are disposable, sealed, blow-moulded, semi-rigid containers made of polyethylene
- Steripods can be poured, used as a dropper or as a syringe to direct the flow of solution; they are an economic alternative to sachets, galley pots, syringes, etc. for wound cleansing

SOFFBAN PLUS (BSN Medical)
- 90% polyester with 10% acrylic fibre containing Triclosan (odour controlling agent)
- synthetic orthopaedic padding which can reduce the risk of unpleasant odours developing under a cast

SOLVALINE N (Lohmann, distributed by Vernon-Carus, DT)
see NON/LOW ADHERENT DRESSINGS
- perforated film, medium absorbency dressing with fast wicking action
- finely perforated 100% polyester fabric cover over a 100% cotton inner
- used for abrasions, lacerations and light to moderately exuding wounds
- fast wicking action to avoid maceration
- 2 non adherent sides to eliminate the risk of placing the dressing 'wrong side down'
- available in sterile and non-sterile dressings

SORBALGON (Hartmann, DT)
see ALGINATE DRESSINGS
- sterile, non-woven dressing of calcium alginate made from marine brown algae
- can be used to cover or lightly fill a wide range of moist wounds, even when infection is present
- available in two square sizes: 5 × 5cm and 10 × 10cm
- **SORBALGON T** tamponade strips are available as 2g/30cm for deep wounds/cavities

SORBSAN (Unomedical, DT)
see ALGINATE DRESSINGS
- sterile dressing of Calcium Alginate BPC derived from seaweed harvested off the coast of West Scotland. This seaweed, *Ascophyllum nodosum*, has a higher mannuronic acid level and produces a soft amorphous gel
- available in three forms :
  - **Flat, surgical dressing** – for shallow wet wounds and ulcers
  - **Surgical packing 2g** – 30cm long for large, deep, open wet wounds
  - **Ribbon 1g** – 40cm long (plus sterile medical probe) – for smaller, deep, open wet wounds; large, wet wound sinuses and wet wounds in awkward locations, e.g. toes and breasts. The probe can be used to assess the extent of the wound size and shape
- may be applied to a wide range of shallow, heavily to medium exuding lesions, even when infection is present[169]
- when in contact with wound secretions containing sodium ions, the insoluble calcium alginate is partially converted to soluble sodium alginate. This forms a hydrophilic gel
- in a clinical comparison of Kaltostat Cavity Dressing and Sorbsan Packing and Ribbon, there was no significant clinical difference in analgesic requirements, mean pain scores or bacterial counts at each dressing change. Nursing staff favoured the handling properties of Sorbsan and its availability in two product sizes[127]

SORBSAN PLUS (Unomedical, DT)
see SORBSAN
- Sorbsan Plus consists of 2 layers :-
  - Sorbsan (calcium alginate) wound contact layer (cream-coloured)
  - Secondary absorbent viscose pad which absorbs excess exudate and wicks laterally

- may be applied to a wide range of shallow, heavily to medium exuding wounds, even when infection is present
- **SORBSAN PLUS CARBON** is available in both non-adhesive and self-adhesive varieties. Contains a carbon fabric which adsorbs odour from the wound exudate. The blue outer layer identifies which way up the dressing should be placed on the wound
- **SORBSAN PLUS NA** is a non-adhesive dressing; the blue outer layer identifies which way up the dressing should be placed on the wound; secured with tape or bandages. Suitable for adhesive allergic patients or for those with fragile skin
- **SORBSAN PLUS SA** is a self-adhesive dressing with a microporous thin foam backing and adhesive; can be used without a secondary dressing; allows patients to shower with dressing in place

SPENCO 2nd SKIN
see PRIMSKIN

SPRAY-ON BIODEGRADABLE FIBRES (Electrosols)
- a spray-on extracellular matrix to help wounds heal without scarring has been developed by Electrosols, a biotechnology company in Haslemere[184]
- spray produces a fine web of biodegradable polymer fibres which encourages growth of fibroblasts and a collagen structure
- not yet tested in humans

SPRILON (S & N)
see AEROSOL SPRAYS, BARRIER FILMS
- an aerosol containing zinc oxide 12.5% and dimeticone 350, 1.04% (CFC free)
- for prophylaxis and treatment of pressure ulcers, moist eczema, skin maceration due to faeces or urine, or around fistulae and ileostomies
- the flexible film formed on the skin allows normal trans-epidermal water loss
- should not be used on patients allergic to wool fat and parabens preservatives

STERI-DRAPE (3M)
see VAPOUR-PERMEABLE FILMS
- polymeric film coated with a hypoallergenic adhesive on one side
- specifically designed as a surgical, adhesive incise drape

STERIFIX (Hartmann, DT)
see NON/LOW-ADHERENT DRESSINGS (similar to Cosmopore E, Medipore, Mepore. Primapore)
- absorbent, perforated dressing with two adhesive border strips
- used for simple wounds and minor injuries with slight exudation

STRAPPAL (S &N, DT))
- a zinc oxide surgical adhesive tape

SUCRALFATE
- non-healing venous stasis ulcers may benefit from the angiogenic activity of topical sucralfate[185]

SUDOCREM (Forest)
see ANTISEPTICS
- an antiseptic emollient cream containing zinc oxide, lanolin (hypo-allergenic), benzyl benzoate, benzylcinnamate and benzyl alcohol
- used to treat pressure ulcers, minor burns and surface wounds
- not recommended as there are blander, less-complex products available

SUGAR PASTE[186]
see HONEY
- sugar has been used for centuries in wound care, e.g., honey to debride wounds and for its antibacterial effects
- thin and thick sugar pastes have been developed at Northwick Park Hospital[187]:

	Thin	Thick
Caster sugar (fine granular sucrose)	1200g	1200g
Icing sugar (additive-free, powdered sucrose)	1800g	1800g
Polyethylene glycol 400	1416ml	686ml
Hydrogen peroxide 30%	23.1ml	19ml

- both pastes are chemically stable for at least six months at 4°C
- additive-free icing sugar can be obtained from Tate and Lyle
- both pastes are used to clean up infected, dirty, malodorous wounds
- thin sugar paste can be instilled into wounds with small openings, using a syringe and quill; thick sugar paste can be moulded with a sterile glove and packed into wounds with a large opening
- twice daily packing of wounds is necessary (or more often)
- some patients find sugar paste dressings painful

- sugar paste lowers the pH of wounds to approximately pH5
- sugar may exert its antibacterial effect by competing for the water present in the cells of bacteria
- Northwick Park has many years' experience of the use of Sugar Paste and has found that even the most offensive wounds are usually fully deodorised within three days; in this respect Sugar Paste is the most effective treatment of "smelly" wounds that they have come across
- sugar is readily available and cheap
- sucrose (a disaccharide of glucose and fructose) if absorbed from a wound, is excreted unchanged in urine
- polyethylene glycol 400 can be absorbed from mucous membranes and high blood levels may be nephrotoxic; sugar paste should be used with care in patients with impaired renal function as any absorbed polyethylene glycol is excreted renally
- sugar paste may cause bleeding when granulation tissue is well formed
- no toxic effects were observed with sugar paste which may be preferable to antiseptics for the management of dirty or infected wounds[188]
- water activity and bacterial growth inhibition have been studied for both sucrose and xylose pastes[189]

SUPERSKIN (Medlogic Global Ltd – distributors, GSL, DT)
see BARRIER FILMS
- a solvent free skin protectant and sealant liquid film containing n-butyl cyanoacrylate
- transparent, waterproof and flexible
- for external use on unbroken skin only to help prevent pressure ulcers and blisters
- can be applied around stomas, wound sites and other areas where skin breakdown is likely to occur e.g. surfaces exposed to friction and shear
- protects skin exposed to irritation from moisture e.g. sweat, urine and digestive juices
- sets within approximately 45 seconds after application
- adheres to skin surface to form a flexible, comfortable barrier
- effective until it wears off naturally by cracking and flaking away as the skin underneath sloughs; re-application may be necessary in 1-3 days
- for single use only – reduces the risk of cross infection
- available as 0.7g (pinpoint accuracy for 10×10cm area) and 2g (for larger areas) applicators

SUPRASORB (Lohmann Rauscher)

- a new range of moist wound dressings consisting of:
  - **Suprasorb A:** calcium alginate dressing and rope
  - **Suprasorb H:** hydrocolloid dressing (standard, thin, sacrum, border))
  - **Suprasorb M:** polyurethane membrane
  - **Suprasorb F:** polyurethane film wound dressing
  - **Suprasorb G:** gel wound dressing and amorphous gel
  - **Suprasorb C:** collagen wound dressing
- none of these are available in the UK except Suprasorb F

SUREPRESS (ConvaTec, DT))

- an elasticated high compression bandage (extensible), type 3c similar to Adva-Co
- incorporates application aids to ensure correct extension and pressure
- can be handwashed in hot soapy water
- **SUREPRESS ABSORBENT PADDING:** a sub-compression wadding bandage used as a component of multi-layer compression bandaging. Protects vulnerable areas and distributes the graduated compression

SURGICEL (J & J)

see HAEMOSTATICS

- sterile, oxidised cellulose which controls bleeding in 2–3 minutes

SURGIPAD (J & J)

- absorbent pad of absorbent cotton and viscose in sleeve of non-woven viscose fabric
- used for heavily exuding wounds requiring frequent dressing changes

SURGISIS (Cook)

- sterile, soft tissue graft
- natural biomaterial harvested from porcine small intestine consisting of a three-dimensional, extracellular matrix comprised of collagen, non-collagenous proteins and other biomolecules
- used as a surgical mesh for implantation to reinforce soft tissue e.g. abdominal wall repair, hernia repair, prolapsed tissue support/repair, general tissue repair
- the body's tissue grows completely into the surgical site while the graft matrix maintains the needed tissue support
- always handle sheets using aseptic technique

- prior to suturing or stapling, ensure that graft is rehydrated with sterile saline or sterile lactated Ringer's solution
- experience indicates that suturing or stapling with close tissue approximation produces better outcomes
- potential complications are: infection, acute or chronic inflammation, allergic reaction
- available in a variety of sizes
- **SURGISIS ES** (enhanced strength): sheets have a thickness and mechanical strength that is several times that of a single layer - designed to tolerate the mechanical stresses associated with higher-stress body systems
- ensure that all layers are secured when suturing or stapling
- **SURGISIS GOLD** (hernia repair graft): sheets have a thickness and mechanical strength that is approximately twice that of Surgisis ES
- **SURGISIS IHM** (inguinal hernia matrix): sheets have a thickness and mechanical strength that is similar to that of Surgisis ES

SYSTEM 4 (Medlock Medical, DT)
see COMPRESSION BANDAGES (FOUR-LAYER)

TAP WATER[190]

- the cleansing of chronic wounds with tap water has not yet been subject to clinical trial but is used in community healthcare
- the infection rate in acute traumatic soft tissue wounds cleaned with tap water was less than that for wounds cleaned with sterile saline; sterile saline should be replaced with tap water[191]
- tap water of drinking quality can be used to irrigate open traumatic wounds[192]
- tap water is as good as sterile saline solution to irrigate simple lacerations prior to repair
- patients may also prefer warmed (to room temperature) tap water for irrigation[193]
- the evidence is limited but one trial suggested that the use of tap water to cleanse acute wounds reduces the infection rate and other trials conclude that there is no difference in the infection and healing rates between wounds that were not cleansed and those cleansed with tap water and other solutions. However the quality of the tap water should be considered prior to its use and in the absence of potable tap water, boiled and cooled water as well as distilled water can be used as wound cleansing agents[194]

TAPELESS PRODUCTS (Mediplus)

- reusable, non-latex dressing holder range
- absorbable stretchable fabric material
- applicable to a wide range of anatomical areas
- Velcro provides quick, reliable, easy to use fastening and adjustment
- fabric material can be customised by cutting without fraying or unravelling
- washable, reusable material using warm water and air drying
- securely positions the primary dressing
- rapid application and removal
- a 'window' allows quick and easy evaluation of the wound site
- no bulk to limit motion of joints

TEGADERM (3M, DT)
see VAPOUR-PERMEABLE FILMS

- consists of a thin polyurethane layer coated with acrylic adhesive
- its unique frame presentation facilitates self-application without causing wrinkling and self-adherence
- may be left in place for up to 10 days
- **TEGADERM HP** (high permeability) dressing – indicated for wounds where moisture accumulation may be a problem
- **TEGADERM IV** dressings – for dressing catheter sites
- **TEGADERM + PAD** combines the features of Tegaderm dressing with an absorbent pad to form an island dressing

TEGAGEN (3M, DT)
see ALGINATE DRESSINGS – formerly called Tegagel

- a non-woven, polysaccharide dressing consisting of condensed fibres of Calcium Alginate BPC derived from pure, natural Scottish seaweed (high concentration of mannuronic acid)
- used for variety of medium to heavily exuding wounds
- wet or dry, the dressing maintains its shape and will not easily pull apart
- can be cut or folded
- may be left in place until saturated or for up to seven days
- **TEGAGEN CAVITY** dressing: 30×2cm rope

TEGAPORE (3M)
see MEMBRANES

- a soft polymer nylon wound contact dressing similar to Urgotul
- made of chemically inert hypoallergenic polyamide net (no adhesive) which is hot rolled to produce a smooth "silk-like" material

- used for partial and full thickness wounds; may also be used on infected wounds
- used as an interface between secondary, absorbent dressing and wound
- does not shed particles or fibres
- pores allow the passage of exudate from moist wounds
- also permeable to topical medicaments and can be used in conjunction with topical agents
- virtually non-adherent
- conforms neatly around difficult to dress bodily areas
- becomes transparent when wet with exudate or saline which allows monitoring of the wound
- can be left in place for extended periods (up to 7 days on clean, exuding wounds) whilst secondary dressings are changed

TEGASORB (3M, DT)
see HYDROCOLLOIDS
- consists of sodium carboxymethylcellulose (CMC) and cross-linked CMC dispersed in a synthetic rubber matrix to give pliability
- border preparation has an outer covering of Tegaderm film extending beyond the hydrocolloid oval – the absorbent mass forms an island in the centre of the film
- used for medium to heavily exuding wounds
- available in bordered oval and non-bordered square shapes
- **TEGASORB THIN (3M, DT)**
  - used for low to medium exuding wounds
  - may be worn for up to 7 days
  - transparent, thin and conformable with optimum absorbency
  - does not contain gelatin or other animal derivatives
  - smooth surface wipes clean and permits bathing
  - available in bordered oval and non-bordered square shapes

TELFA (Tyco Healthcare, DT)
see NON/LOW ADHERENT DRESSINGS (similar to Cutilin, Interpose, Melolin, Release, Skintact, Solvaline N)
- absorbent, perforated plastic film faced dressing
- consists of a thin layer of absorbent cotton fibres enclosed in a perforated sleeve
- ideal for lightly exuding wounds
- can be cut to fit any shape without separating
- **TELFA PLUS:** super absorbent pad
- **TELFA MAX:** ultra-absorbent pad

- **TELFA ISLAND:** absorbent, perforated dressing with adhesive border (similar to Cosmopor E, Medipore, Mepore, Primapore, Sterifix)

TELFA CLEAR (Tyco Healthcare)
- a non-adherent, non-absorbent dressing consisting of a polyester mylar film
- used in burns, skin grafts and donor sites, abrasions, surgical incisions and chronic wounds
- can be used with ointments
- available as sterile dressings and a non-sterile bulk roll

TENDERWET (Hartmann)
- a multi-layer wound dressing pad containing a superabsorbent polyacrylate core with irrigating properties as its central component
- used for wound cleansing when wet therapy is needed
- while it is still in its package, the dressing is activated before use with an appropriate volume of Ringer's solution which is then delivered continuously to the wound for up to 24 hours. This actively softens and detaches necrotic tissue. The absorbent core takes up and retains micro-organisms and wound exudate. These two actions simultaneously rinse and cleanse the wound
- upper moisture repellent layer prevents strike through of the dressing
- dressings should be changed once daily
- **Tenderwet 24** delivers set volumes of Ringer's Solution for about 24 hours and therefore should be changed daily. Has a moisture repellent layer beneath the top layer
- **Tenderwet Standard** delivers set volumes of Ringer's Solution for about 12 hours and therefore should be changed twice daily. This does not have an upper moisture repellent layer. Particularly suitable for deep wounds
- both dressings are available in 4 different sizes and shapes (but not yet in the Drug Tariff)

TERRA-CORTRIL (Pfizer, POM)
- 1% hydrocortisone/3% oxytetracycline ointment
- used widely by plastic surgeons for hypertrophic, oedematous granulating wounds
- commonly believed that steroids have a direct action in decreasing the size and porosity of the granulations which allows the antibiotic access to the fine spaces between the granulation tissue
- should only be used sparingly for a short period

TIELLE (J & J, DT)
see FOAMS
- a particulate-free, synthetic hydropolymer; island dressing consisting of:
  - a waterproof, permeable, polyurethane backing which acts as a barrier to micro-organisms and has a skin-friendly adhesive
  - non-woven wicking layer (fluid transport) which draws exudate from the hydropolymer, allowing it to evaporate through the outer layer
  - highly absorbent hydropolymer central island which expands as exudate is taken up
- a hydropolymer is a non-particulate polymer or mixture of polymers, the polymers being hydrophilic and interactive with aqueous fluids
- does not liquefy or breakdown and therefore leaves no particulate matter in the wound
- in a randomised controlled clinical study comparing Tielle with Granuflex, Tielle was better in preventing leakage and reducing odour, but there were no differences in healing rates of patients with leg ulcers or pressure ulcers[87]
- provides a moist healing environment which allows granulation to proceed under optimum conditions
- used for low to medium exuding wounds
- should not be used on clinically infected wounds without medical supervision
- does not require a secondary dressing
- suitable for use under compression bandaging
- may be left *in situ* for up to 7 days depending on exudate levels
- available as square, rectangular and sacral dressings with adhesive borders
- **TIELLE BORDERLESS:** square dressings without adhesive border

TIELLE LITE (J & J, DT)
see FOAMS and TIELLE
- a sterile, polyurethane, foam, film dressing
- the inner surface of the polyurethane foam island is covered with an apertured plastic film made from ethyl methyl acrylate that acts as a low-adherent wound contact layer and reduces loss of fluid by evaporation
- used for dry to low exuding wounds
- available as square and rectangular dressings with borders

TIELLE PACKING (J & J, DT)
see FOAMS, TIELLE
- a hydropolymer cavity dressing
- highly absorbent and gently expands as it takes up exudate

- used for medium to heavily exuding cavity wounds e.g. chronic and deep wounds
- not used on third degree burns, lesions with active vasculitis or infected wounds
- may be left in place for 7 days depending upon the amount of exudate

TIELLE PLUS (J & J, DT)
see FOAMS and TIELLE
- a sterile, polyurethane foam, film dressing similar to Tielle
- indicated for medium to heavily exuding wounds
- has a superabsorbent wicking layer able to absorb up to 300 times its own weight
- available as square, rectangular and sacral dressings with adhesive borders
- **TIELLE PLUS BORDERLESS:** square and rectangular dressings without adhesive border

TISEPT (Medlock Medical)
see CHLORHEXIDINE, CETRIMIDE
- contains chlorhexidine gluconate (0.015%) and cetrimide (0.15%) in a clear yellow aqueous solution
- not recommended for wound care because of cetrimide content

TOPIGEL (Inamed)
- a soft, slightly adhesive, semi-occlusive polyester fabric reinforced gel sheet
- used to treat keloid and hypertrophic scarring

TRANSORBENT (Unomedical, DT)
see FOAMS (formerly called Askina Transorbent)
- adhesive polyurethane foam film dressing consisting of 5 layers:
  - water-based adhesive
  - non-adherent wound contact fabric
  - hydrogel layer
  - foam layer
  - film layer
- used for light to medium exuding wounds
- may be left in place for up to 7 days before changing
- available as square and rectangular dressings (without borders)

TRENTAL (Aventis Pharma, POM)
see PENTOXIFYLLINE

TRICOTEX (S & N, DT)
see NON/LOW ADHERENT DRESSINGS
- a sterile, knitted viscose primary dressing

TRIONIC (Laboratoire Brothier, DT)
see ALGINATE DRESSINGS
- contains calcium alginate, zinc and manganese ions (trace elements) and chlorophyllin which gives the dressing its green colour
- available as:
  - plain dressings suitable for medium to heavily exuding wounds
  - a rope dressing for medium to heavily exuding cavities
- can be used on many different types of wounds – superficial, deep, acute, chronic infected
- Haddenham Healthcare Ltd are the distributors in the UK

TRUFOAM (Unomedical, DT)
see FOAMS
- a polyurethane foam film dressing with or without an adhesive border similar to Biatain Adhesive, Lyofoam Extra Adhesive and Tielle
- consists of a highly absorbent hydrophilic foam pad, covered with a flesh-coloured, microporous, thin-foam backing
- used for medium exuding, partial or full thickness wounds
- the foam will expand as it absorbs exudate to fill and conform to wound cavities
- not recommended for dry superficial wounds
- can be left in place for up to 7 days depending on exudate levels
- available as:
- **TRUFOAM SA** self-adhesive dressing; the backing extends to provide an adhesive border; particularly useful on more mobile patients
- **TRUFOAM NA** non-adhesive dressing; particularly useful with adhesive-allergic patients or those with fragile skin; applied white side down and secured with tape or bandages

TULLE (MEDICATED) DRESSINGS
see BACTIGRAS, INADINE, M AND M
- used for infected, superficial wounds
- do not provide an ideal wound healing environment

- on the basis of evidence available to date, it appears that chlorhexidine tulle gras is the superior product[195]

TULLE (NON-MEDICATED) DRESSINGS
see ATRAUMAN, PARAFFIN GAUZE/TULLE GRAS (NON-MEDICATED), VASELINE PETROLATUM
- do not provide an ideal wound healing environment

ULTEC PRO (Tyco Healthcare, DT)
see HYDROCOLLOIDS
- consists of gel-forming polymers with 30% alginate and a polyurethane film backing
- used for light to medium exuding wounds
- available with and without an adhesive border (thin profile) and as sacral dressings

ULTRA FOUR NON-LATEX BANDAGES (Robinson Healthcare, DT))
see COMPRESSION BANDAGES (FOUR-LAYER)

UNISEPT (Medlock Medical)
see ANTISEPTICS and CHLORHEXIDINE
- contains chlorhexidine gluconate (0.05% w/v) in a clear, pink aqueous solution
- available in 25ml and 100ml sterile sachets
- used for cleansing and disinfecting wounds and burns

UNITULLE (Aventis, DT)
see PARAFFIN GAUZE/TULLE GRAS
- a "light loaded" sterile product containing 90 to 130g of paraffin base per square metre of cloth
- is contra-indicated where there is known allergy to lanolin

URGOSORB (Parema, DT)
see ALGINATES and HYDROCOLLOIDS
- a combination dressing of hydrocolloid particles (sodium carboxymethylcellulose) and calcium alginate fibres
- used for medium to heavily exuding acute and chronic wounds
- can be used on infected wounds (changed daily) and for haemostasis
- requires a secondary dressing
- may be left in place for up to 7 days depending on the level of exudate

- **URGOSORB ROPE:** cavity dressing – pack loosely without excessive pressure

URGOTUL (Parema, DT)
see HYDROCOLLOIDS
- soft polymer wound contact dressing
- a hydrocolloid dressing consisting of a textile net impregnated with hydrocolloid particles dispersed in a lipophilic matrix of petroleum gel. This mass contains carboxymethylcellulose, paraffin, petroleum jelly and carrier polymers
- the impregnated aerated net is non-greasy to the touch, thin, pliable and conformable
- on contact with wound exudate, the hydrocolloid particles form a gel and interact with the petroleum gel component to form a lipido-colloid interface with the wound
- used to treat acute and chronic wounds in the granulation and epithelialisation stage
- can be cut to shape of the wound
- requires a secondary dressing; with an exuding wound, the open mesh structure allows exudate to drain through to the secondary dressing
- when compared to traditional greasy tulle dressings, Urgotul is non-adherent which allows non-traumatic removal
- adheres to latex surgical gloves (moisten gloves with normal saline to facilitate handling)
- change every 2-3 days (depending on the wound)

URGOTUL SSD (Parema, DT)
see ANTIBACTERIALS, HYDROCOLLOIDS, SILVER, URGOTUL
- soft polymer wound contact dressing impregnated with silver sulfadiazine
- polyester mesh impregnated with hydrocolloid particles (carboxymethylcellulose), petroleum jelly and silver sulfadiazine (3.75%)
- used for superficial or deep 2nd degree burns where there is a risk of infection
- change every 24-48 hours but may be left on for up to 5 days depending on wound conditions
- requires a secondary dressing
- treatment should be limited to not more than one month

VACUTEX (Protex Capillary Dressings Ltd., DT)
- a non-woven, low-adherent, occlusive capillary dressing which is very absorbent (similar to Advadraw)
- consists of 2 outer polyester layers sandwiching a polyester cotton core

- works by capillary action, drawing exudate away from the wound site into the cotton core, thereby creating a clean wound environment and reducing potential maceration
- in cavity wounds, dressing is cut to the size and shape of the wound; in superficial wounds, there is no need to cut to shape
- in exuding wounds, the dressing is applied in multiple layers, to enable larger volumes of exudate to be absorbed, to avoid leakage or strike through
- has the ability to manage medium to high levels of exudate and promotes debridement of necrotic and sloughy wounds
- unsuitable for use near arterial wounds or severely painful wounds
- an independent audit demonstrated a high patient acceptability as measured by improvement in the wound, comfort, nursing ease of use and odour reduction. The diversity of wound types and locations were treated successfully with the potential to be cost-effective[196]

VACUUM-ASSISTED CLOSURE (VAC) THERAPY (KCI Medical)

- the VAC unit applies negative pressure to a specialised dressing positioned in the wound cavity or over a flap or graft. Excess fluid is collected in a disposable canister
- helps to reduce oedema, increase blood supply and decrease bacterial colonisation
- the therapy has proven to be effective with cardiothoracic surgical wounds[197], pressure ulcers, chronic wounds and grafts
- VAC is a useful adjunctive therapy for the management of a wide variety of wounds. It can be used to promote rapid granulation, reduce bacterial colonisation and manage exudate[198]

VAPOUR-PERMEABLE FILMS

see ACTIVHEAL, ALLDRESS, ARGLAES, BIOCLUSIVE, BLISTERFILM, CENTRAL GARD, C-VIEW, DERMAFILM, EasI-V, ENSURE-IT, EPI-FIX, HYDROFILM, IOBAN-II, IV3000, MEFILM, MEPORE ULTRA, NIKO-FIX, OPRAFLEX, OPSITE, POLYSKIN II, (POLYVINYLCHLORIDE), STERIDRAPE, SUPRASORB F, TEGADERM

- sterile, thin, conformable, vapour-permeable, hypoallergenic adhesive-coated films with or without an absorbent backing
- only considered suitable for relatively shallow wounds with low amounts of exudate e.g., dermabrasion, burns and donor sites. Also used prophylactically to protect vulnerable areas of skin, to prevent pressure ulcers, as retention dressings, e.g., for cannulas and in theatres for operative surgery (as sterile drapes)

- are not suitable for patients with thin, friable skin as they may cause damage on removal
- probably the single most important feature of films is their ability to permit the passage of water vapour from beneath the film to the external environment (moisture-vapour transmission rate, MVTR) (199). The MVTR will be compromised if used in combination with other dressings (applies to all dressings having a MVTR)
- the skin around the wound needs to be clean and dry prior to application of the film
- on removal, most films may be stretched parallel with the skin to break the adhesive which allows removal without trauma
- are supported on a removable carrier that assists in the application of the dressing
- are variably transparent, depending on the product enabling monitoring of skin and wound
- have many of the characteristics of an ideal dressing (*see* appendix) except:
  - excessive exudate may accumulate under the dressing. This is often aspirated using a sterile syringe – the puncture hole being covered with a small piece of the film. However, it is better practice to remove the film and apply a new dressing. This prevents infecting the wound and eliminates needle-stick injuries;
  - the film may cling to itself during application and may need considerable skill to apply e.g. two pairs of hands;
  - may be some adhesive trauma on removal, especially on inflamed, fragile skin;
  - they cool the surface of the wound
- patients can bathe or shower as vapour-permeable films are waterproof
- can stay in place for up to 7 days depending on exudate production; may be left in place for longer than 7 days if being used on intact skin for pressure ulcer prophylaxis
- the properties of six semi-permeable film dressings have been compared[200]
- a meta-analysis shows that there is a significantly increased risk of catheter-tip infection with the use of transparent dressings compared with gauze dressings when used with either central or peripheral catheters[201]
- the Cochrane Review has been updated[202]. There is a high level of uncertainty regarding the risk of infection with central venous catheter dressings (gauze and tape or transparent polyurethane films). It appears that the choice of dressing for central venous catheters can be based on patient preference. Further randomised controlled trials are necessary

128

VARIDASE TOPICAL (Wyeth, POM)[203]

- sterile dry powder containing two enzymes, streptokinase and streptodornase, which is stored in the refrigerator (2–8°C.)
- Varidase Topical Combi-Pack includes a vial of Varidase powder, a 20ml flip-top vial of sterile normal saline (diluent), a sterile transfer needle and full instructions on the method of reconstitution
- needs to be reconstituted with 20ml sterile sodium chloride 0.9% w/v solution (stable for up to 24 hours stored in a refrigerator at 2–8°C). Do not shake the vial vigorously when reconstituting otherwise the enzymes will be denatured
- used for cleansing of necrotic and infected wounds and suppurative surface lesions
- needs to be applied once or twice a day and may be covered by a film dressing
- allergic reactions may occur infrequently
- streptokinase degrades fibrin and fibrinogen; streptodornase liquefies and facilitates the removal of DNA derived from cell nuclei. This facilitates cleansing and desloughing of the wound
- as Varidase does not contain a preservative, multi-dose use is not recommended
- can be injected by experienced staff under dry scabs or applied on the surfaces of scabs which have been cross-hatched with a sterile scalpel
- in a randomised, double-blind, controlled trial, a comparison was made of the relative efficacy of using Varidase in KY Jelly or KY Jelly alone. The results suggest that KY Jelly may be a cost effective alternative to the use of Varidase in KY Jelly[128]
- patients treated with topical Varidase all showed an increase in antistreptokinase titres. It would therefore seem prudent to restrict the use of topical streptokinase to patients not at risk of myocardial infarction[204]
- topical streptokinase causes a significant humoral response by one month, which then declines. To ensure thrombolytic efficacy, therefore, it may be preferable to avoid intravenous streptokinase in patients who have been treated with topical streptokinase in the preceding six months[205]
- the vial only presentation was discontinued due to minimal use in the UK

VARIHESIVE (ConvaTec)
see HYDROCOLLOIDS
- wafers containing gelatin 20%, pectin 20%, polyisobutylene 40%, sodium carboxymethylcellulose 20%
- European equivalent of Granuflex

VASELINE PETROLATUM GAUZE (Tyco Healthcare)
see TULLE NON-MEDICATED
- fine mesh, absorbent gauze impregnated with white petrolatum
- used on dry to light exuding wounds
- available as strips in tubes or foil packs

VELBAND (J & J, DT)
- sub-compression absorbent wadding bandage

VERSIVA (ConvaTec, DT)
see HYDROCOLLOIDS
- a hydrocolloid dressing with an adhesive border consisting of a:
  - wound contact layer of thin, perforated hydrocolloid adhesive (holds the dressing in place and allows fast absorption of exudate)
  - non-woven fibrous hydrofibre layer (adsorbs and retains exudate by forming a cohesive gel)
  - viscous material (wicks fluid away)
  - top polyurethane foam-film layer (protects the wound and allows moisture vapour transmission of exudate)
- acts as a barrier to the wound against bacterial, viral and external contamination
- used as a primary dressing for moderately exuding wounds
- used as a secondary dressing with Aquacel to manage more heavily exuding wounds
- maximum recommended wear time is 7 days
- available in square, rectangular, heel and sacral shapes

VIDENE (Adams)
see ANTISEPTICS and POVIDONE-IODINE
- 10% antiseptic solution for pre-operative skin disinfection and general antisepsis

WOUND DRAINAGE POUCHES
see BIOTROL DRAINA S FISTULA, CONVATEC WOUND MANAGER and OAKMED OPTION WOUND MANAGER

YOGHURT
- made from milk which has been heat-treated and then inoculated with harmless bacteria, e .g. *Streptococcus thermophilus, Lactobacillus bulgaricus* or *Lactobacillus acidophilus*

- after the bacteria have multiplied, the mixture is chilled (2 weeks' expiry) or pasteurised (3 months' expiry)
- wound healing folk-lore describes the use of yoghurt but scientific proof is required
- can be used twice daily for three days, then daily
- soothing but messy

ZINC
see CURASORB ZN and ZINC SULPHATE
- a systematic literature review has shown that oral zinc sulphate does not appear to aid healing of leg ulcers, although it might be beneficial in those with venous leg ulcers and a low serum zinc. Further research is needed to verify this and if so to ascertain the serum zinc concentration below which treatment with zinc is beneficial, and to ascertain the optimum treatment regimen[206]

ZINC SULPHATE LOTION (Lotio Rubra)
- Zinc sulphate 1%, with amaranth, in water
- apply undiluted as a wet dressing

ZIPZOC (S & N)
- a sterile rayon stocking impregnated with 20% zinc oxide ointment and no preservatives
- used for treatment of chronic leg ulcers and chronic venous insufficiency
- applied from the base of the toes to below the knee
- can be used as the primary contact layer and under compression bandaging
- should be changed at least weekly
- not as absorbent as paste bandages – exudate passes through stocking into a secondary pad
- one size comfortably fits legs 14 to 60cm in circumference
- to protect clothes from Zipzoc, a suitable outer bandage should be worn
- a licensed medicine and is available on NHS prescription, however it is not a medical device and therefore will not appear under section IXA of the DT

MANAGEMENT OF WOUNDS/ WOUND TYPES[207, 208]

ARTERIAL WOUNDS
- a precise diagnosis is required[209]
- assess causative and contributive factors e.g. to differentiate between arterial, venous and mixed aetiologies
- address any risk factors, pain (at rest or nocturnal), pressure and friction, history of the wound, medications, nutritional status etc.
- determine perfusion status, pulse status, ankle brachial index, arterial occlusive disease, ischaemia, wound characteristics and complications
- consider surgical options e.g. bypass surgery, amputation
- debridement may be contraindicated in arterial wounds
- paste bandages are used to treat skin conditions
- compression bandages are contraindicated
- promote exercise according to tolerability
- promote smoking cessation
- Radiometer has introduced a new, cost-effective, multi-channel transcutaneous oxygen monitor. This enables accurate mapping of tissue oxygenation and perfusion in patients with non-healing limb wounds or other types of peripheral vascular disease. Further information is available on: www.radiometer.com/wounds

BURNS AND SCALDS[210]
- ABC of burns: a series of 12 articles in a BMJ clinical review provides an overview of the most important aspects of burn injuries for hospital and non-hospital healthcare workers[211]
- burns are classified into 2 groups by the amount of skin loss[211]:
  - partial thickness burns do not extend through all skin layers
    * superficial – an epidermal burn e.g. sunburn
    * superficial dermal – epidermis and upper layers of dermis e.g. blistering
    * deep dermal – epidermis and deeper layers of dermis but not entire dermis
  - full thickness burns extend through all skin layers into the subcutaneous tissues
- the main aims of burn care are to restore form, function and feeling
- burn management consists of 7 stages – rescue, resuscitate, retrieve,

resurface, rehabilitate, reconstruct and review
- cooling with tepid tap water (10–15 minutes) is one of the most important first aid measures
- simple dressings are used such as non-medicated paraffin tulles, Flamazine
- pain relief will be required because of exposed nerve endings
- routine use of antibiotics should be discouraged
- HF-Antidote Gel is used for hydrofluoric acid burns

CARE OF SKIN SURROUNDING WOUNDS
- Paste bandages (depending on the state of the skin)

CAVITY WOUNDS[212, 213]
- cavity wounds should not be packed tightly or over-filled
- there are a variety of products available:
  - Foams: Allevyn Cavity Wound Dressing; Cavi-Care, Tielle
  - Alginate: rope, ribbon, cavity dressings
  - Hydroactives: Allevyn Plus Cavity
  - Hydrogels: gel products;
  - Hydrocolloids: pastes/gels, Contreet
  - Sugar pastes: thin and thick

  - Iodoflex
  - Iodosorb ointment $\left.\right\}$ infected cavities

CELLULITIS
- anatomical features, manifestations, initiating sources of infection, differential diagnosis, antimicrobial treatment, clinical recommendations and guidelines have been reviewed by Swartz[214]

DIABETIC ULCERS[215-220]
- a precise diagnosis is required
- management principles are:
  - share decision making between patient and professional
  - ongoing care should involve recall and annual review
  - examine for risk factors for ulceration
  - test foot sensation and foot pulses
  - inspect for foot deformity and footwear
  - classify foot risk as: at low current risk, at increased risk, at high risk, ulcerated foot
  - treat any infection

- establish whether any associated ischaemia is amenable to revascularisation
- keep forces applied to the ulcerated area to a minimum
- improve the condition of the wound
- consider prevention of ulcer recurrence
- there is evidence of effectiveness of the following for prevention:
  - identification of those at high risk
  - referral to foot care clinics which offer education, podiatry and footwear
  - therapeutic shoes with custom-moulded insoles
  - NICE has recently published a clinical guideline on the prevention and management of foot problems[221]
- the following treatments may be beneficial but further trials are required:
  - total contact casting
  - growth factors e.g. Regranex
  - G-CSF for patients with severe infections
  - 2% ketanserin ointment
  - Iamin ointment
  - debridement with cadexomer iodine
  - Dermagraft
  - there is some evidence that people with diabetic foot ulcers are less likely to have a major amputation if they receive hyperbaric oxygen therapy. This is based on 3 randomised trials with a limited number of patients. Further research is required[152]
- the NICE appraisal of new treatments has been withdrawn from the work programme and incorporated into the NICE clinical guidelines on wound care management
- diabetics with risk factors require more frequent monitoring. Patients with sensory loss require regular podiatric care and should be educated regarding preventative foot care e.g. wearing shoes with adequate depth and width. Non-infected neuropathic foot ulcers require debridement and reduction of pressure. Ulcers with signs of clinical infection require sharp debridement and systemic antibiotics guided by appropriate cultures. Continuous use of the antibiotic until the ulcer has healed is not recommended[222]

DIGITAL ULCERS
- Bosentan (Tracleer) can be used to treat ulcers that form on the fingers in scleroderma (reported at the annual meeting of the American College of Rheumatology in Florida on 26 October 2003). Bosentan is an endothelin receptor antagonist. High levels of endothelin can cause vasoconstriction, fibrosis and inflammation

DISCOLOURED, UNBROKEN SKIN
- dry skin: simple bland ointments e.g. yellow/white soft paraffin
- skin conditions associated with wounds: paste bandages
- skin subject to pressure or trauma: non-adhesive dressings, foam dressings; low-adherent dressings; non-medicated tulles; vapour-permeable films

DONOR SITES[223]
- partial-dermal thickness wounds are left to heal by secondary intention
- pain/discomfort and exudate are the main concerns for management
- appropriate dressings are:
  - hydrocolloids
  - alginates
  - hydrofibres
  - foams
  - semi-permeable films
  - silicones

EPITHELIALISING WOUNDS
- dressing choice depends on level of exudate
- vapour-permeable films; membranes; paraffin tulle
- hydrocolloids; hydrogels
- alginates; foams
- low-adherent dressings

EXUDING WOUNDS[224-226]
- the purpose of exudate is to maintain a moist wound environment without causing maceration
- exudate consists of serum without blood cells and has a high protein content. It also contains nutrients and inflammatory components
- elevation of the leg and compression bandaging are important elements of treatment to reduce exudate in venous ulceration
- levels of exudate are often described as light, medium or heavy and this influences the choice of dressing used:
  - None-light exudate
    * Foams   Cavi-Care, Flexipore
    * Hydrogel: Actiformcool, Aquaform, Intrasite
  - Light-medium exudate
    * Foams: Biatain, Lyofoam
    * Alginates: Curasorb
    * Hydrocolloids: transparent/thin dressings; Combiderm, Hydrocoll

    * Hydrogel: Aquaflo, wet Geliperm
    * Hydroactives: Allevyn Thin
 – Medium – heavy exudate
    * Alginates: Algisite M, Algosteril. Sorbsan
    * Hydrocolloids: Alione, Aquacel, Hydrocoll
    * Foams: Activheal, Hydrafoam, Tielle Plus
    * Hydroactives: Allevyn Compression, Cutinova Hydro
    * Advadraw, Drawtex, Eclypse
 – Heavy exudate
    * Algosteril, Allevyn, Lyofoam Extra, Mesalt, Seasorb Soft, Sorbsan
      Plus, Vacutex
    * Wound drainage pouches

FLAT, DRY WOUNDS
- low-adherent dressings; vapour-permeable films; membranes

FLAT, MOIST WOUNDS
- low-adherent dressings; non-medicated tulles; vapour-permeable films;
- membranes; hydrocolloids; hydrogels; foams; alginates

GRANULATING WOUNDS
- dressing choice depends on level of exudate and depth of wound
- hydrocolloids; alginates; foams; hydrogels, silicone dressings

INFECTED WOUNDS[227, 228]
- the clinical criteria for wound infection are identified for acute and surgical wounds, diabetic foot ulcers, venous and arterial leg ulcers, pressure ulcers and burns[229]
- the key principles for the management of a patient with a wound infection are[230]:
  - treat the patient holistically
  - recognise the signs of inflammation/increased burden/clinical infection
  - be able to take 'reliable' wound swabs
  - be able to interpret culture reports
  - treat the infection - causative organism(s) – consider antibiotic sensitivities
  - consider which wound management products are suitable and appropriate
  - minimize the risk of cross infection
  - reduce the risk of any complications
  - educate the patient and his/her family and carers

- prevention of wound infection should be a primary aim
- the classic signs of wound infection are localised erythema, localised pain, localised heat, cellulitis and oedema
- the 'wound infection continuum' extends from sterility to infection:
  - sterility (absence of microbes)
    * no treatment for infection
  - contamination (presence of microbes but little active growth) is treated by:
    * general infection control measures e.g. hand washing
  - colonisation (growth and death of microbes is kept at a safe level by host immune response) and is treated by:
    * general infection control measures e.g. hand washing (which do not disturb the balance)
  - critical colonisation (host defences are unable to maintain a balance between the number of bacteria and the defence systems available) is treated by:
    * debridement if appropriate
    * antiseptics e.g. restrict to chlorhexidine and povidone-iodine products
  - infection (host defences overwhelmed) is treated by:
    * systemic antibiotics – depending on local/systemic signs of infection
    * antibacterials e.g. Flamazine
    * +/– antiseptics

MALIGNANT/FUNGATING WOUNDS

- are a distressing problem for a significant number of patients with advanced cancer
- the goal of care is to maintain or improve quality of life through symptom control[231]
- control bleeding
- assess pain and analgesia requirements
- treat or mask odour
- debride wound
- reduce volume of exudate
- reduce inflammation e.g. by removing sensitising agents
- care for surrounding skin
- improve cosmetic appearance e.g. reduce tumour bulk; avoid bulky dressings
- enable patient to cope with altered body image
- provide palliative care[232]

MALODOROUS WOUNDS
- an offensive or "smelly" wound is usually associated with anaerobic activity
- reducing levels of bacterial colonisation is the most effective way of managing malodorous wounds
  - systemic antibiotics/antimicrobials
  - larval therapy e.g. LarvE, BioBags
  - metronidazole gels – use judiciously e.g. for fungating, malodorous tumours only
  - honey or sugar paste (thick and thin)
  - odour absorbing dressings e.g. activated charcoal dressings
- complementary therapies or air fresheners are used to mask the smell

NECROTIC WOUNDS[233-235]
- debridement enables the removal of dead tissue, cell debris or foreign bodies from a wound e.g black heel, and is essential if wound healing is to proceed
- dry necrotic tissue (eschar) is black and leathery in appearance – as moisture content increases, the colour changes to brown, yellow or grey
- evidence is lacking about the best way to debride. The main methods are:
  - Modern products promote autolysis:
    * hydrogels e.g. gel products, Intrasite Conformable
    * hydrocolloids e.g. paste/gels
    * alginates
    * sugar pastes (thick and thin)
    * sodium chloride 0.9% w/v irrigation
  - Sharp debridement
    * surgical (using a scalpel/scissors with a local/general anaesthetic)
    * conservative (at the bedside)
  - Biosurgical debridement using larvae e.g. LarvE, BioBag
  - Mechanical debridement
    * wet-to-dry saline-soaked gauze
    * compression therapy
    * whirlpool, hydrotherapy, high pressure irrigation, pulsed lavage
  - Enzymatic debridement e.g. Varidase, bacterial-derived collagenases
  - Chemical e.g. chlorinated solutions, hydrogen peroxide. These delay wound healing and irritate the surrounding skin so should not be used
- debridement treatments are risky and practitioners using sharp debridement should complete specific training before undertaking the procedure[233, 234]

OEDEMATOUS WOUNDS
- use compression bandages; exercise; elevation of leg

- use intermittent sequential compression therapy[236]

OVER/HYPERGRANULATION TISSUE
see SCAR MANAGEMENT
- occurs in many types of wounds when the inflammatory phase of healing is prolonged unnecessarily
- ideally any treatment should not further exacerbate the inflammatory reaction and should be non-traumatic
- there is no consensus as to the correct treatment but the most frequently used methods are[237]:
  - change from an occlusive to a non-occlusive dressing such as Lyofoam[238]
  - application of light pressure to the wound bed by the addition of supplementary padding e.g. silicone dressings
  - short-term application of a low dose of corticosteroid e.g. Terracortril (tetracycline and hydrocortisone ointment) or Daktacort (miconazole and hydrocortisone cream) – not ideal
  - removal using a caustic substance such as silver nitrate sticks/compresses – not ideal
  - allowing the hypergranulation to resolve itself without treatment
- other less ideal treatments are currettage, cautery, phenol and polysporin

PRESSURE ULCERS
- formerly known as pressure sores, bed sores and decubitus ulcers
- damage to the skin is caused by extrinsic factors (pressure, shearing forces, friction) and intrinsic forces (illness, age, nutritional status, drug therapy)
- the toes, heels, sacrum and ischial tuberosities are most at risk of developing pressure ulcers
- the principles of pressure ulcer management and prevention have been reviewed by the Wound Care Society[239]
- NICE has published several articles on pressure ulcer risk assessment and prevention:
  - a clinical guideline[240]
  - a guide for patients and their carers:[241]
  - equipment selection:[242]
- the RCN has published a guide to assist in the implementation of national guidelines[243]
- the evidence of the effects of dressings is poor[244]
- psychoactive drugs may have a role in pressure sore origin[245]
- topical application of nerve growth factor may be an effective therapy for patients with severe pressure ulcers of the foot[246]. An editorial notes that the

data were somewhat limited by the design of this randomised, double-blind, placebo-controlled trial
- a recent updated review found that it was not possible to draw any firm conclusions on the effect of enteral and parenteral nutrition on the prevention and treatment of pressure ulcers. Further trials of high methodological quality are necessary[247]
- the European Pressure Ulcer Advisory Panel (www.epuap.org):
  – has produced treatment and prevention guidance for pressure ulcers
  – will launch the final version of its guideline on nutrition in pressure ulcer prevention and treatment at the World Union of Wound Healing Societies meeting in Paris in July 2004

RECALCITRANT WOUNDS
- a precise diagnosis is required
- growth factors
- skin substitutes e.g. Apligraf, Biobrane, Dermagraft, Integra, Oasis
- hyalofill

SCAR MANAGEMENT[248]
- the main types of scars are:
  – mature scars - flat and light coloured;
  – immature scars -red, sometimes itchy or painful, slightly elevated;
  – linear hypertrophic scars e.g. surgical/traumatic;
  – widespread hypertrophic scars e.g. burn;
  – keloids - minor and major
- it is much more efficient to prevent hypertrophic scars than to treat them. The consensus is that the most successful treatment of a hypertrophic scar or keloid is achieved when the scar is immature but the overlying epithelium is intact.
- the risk of scarring is reduced by good surgical technique and wound management. In addition, scarring can be prevented by:
  – low risk - silicone gel sheeting;
  – increased risk - hypoallergenic taping or silicone gel sheeting;
  – high risk - silicone gel sheeting
  – concurrent intralesional corticosteroid injections as second-line prophylaxis for more severe cases;
- there are other therapies in common use, however, further evidence is required of efficacy:
  – pressure therapy;
  – radiotherapy;

- laser therapy;
- cryotherapy
- there is emerging evidence of efficacy for:
  - interferons;
  - intralesional 5-fluorouracil;
  - bleomycin injections
  - initial trials of Transforming Growth Factor beta 3 that reduces scar formation have produced encouraging results. It acts by speeding up cell migration which allows the skin to regenerate its usual orderly structure before a scar can form[249]

SKIN GRAFTS[250]
see DURASIS and SURGISIS
- different types known as:
  - autographs – taken from patient's own uninjured skin or grown from patient's skin cells into a dressing;
  - allographs – applied as a sheet of bioengineered skin grown from donor cells;
  - xerographs – preserved skin from other animals e.g. pigs
- there is limited evidence that artificial skin used in conjunction with compression bandaging, increases the chance of healing a venous ulcer compared with compression alone

SLOUGHY WOUNDS[251–253]
- slough is yellow or grey, stringy tissue that adheres to the wound bed and resembles the appearance and texture of mozzarella cheese on a pizza. It should not be confused with the yellow gelatinous coating of fibrin which is occasionally seen resembling melted cheese on toast[234]
- optimum healing will not occur until the slough is removed. The main methods of removing slough are described under **NECROTIC WOUNDS**

SURGICAL WOUNDS
- there is insufficient evidence to suggest whether the choice of dressing or topical agent affects the healing of surgical wounds healing by secondary intention although gauze may be associated with greater pain or discomfort for the patient[254]

VENOUS/ARTERIAL ULCERS
- a precise diagnosis is required[209]
- as for arterial ulcers except that reduced compression may be indicated under medical supervision (ABPI 0.6-0.7)

VENOUS ULCERS[255–256]

- American authors have reviewed the management of patients with venous ulcers[257]
- a precise diagnosis is required to eliminate other possible causes e.g. arterial insufficiency, neuropathy
- use of graduated compression is the cornerstone of therapy
- in a randomised controlled comparison of surgery and compression with compression alone, surgical correction of superficial venous reflux reduces 12-month ulcer recurrence. Most patients with chronic venous ulceration will benefit from compression and the addition of simple venous surgery[258]
- elevation of the limb and exercise (improving mobility) are also important (within specialist-nurse led clinics)
- reducing obesity and improving nutrition are effective treatments
- selected patients may require skin grafting or venous surgery
- paste bandages are used to treat skin conditions surrounding the wound
- pneumatic compression therapy for venous insufficiency may be useful but further trials are required (*see* PNEUMATIC COMPRESSION)
- the NICE appraisal of new treatments has been withdrawn from the work programme and incorporated into the NICE clinical guidelines on wound care management
- community leg ulcer clinics using compression bandaging have dramatically improved healing rates and reduced costs, but close supervision by leg ulcer nurse specialists is essential if standards are to be maintained. Future research should focus on preventing ulceration by identifying at risk populations[259]

DISCONTINUED PRODUCTS

Algistat
Askina Biofilm S
Askina Jet Saline
Askina Spray Aerosol
Aserbine cream
Bard Absorption Dressing
Boric acid lint
Chlorasol
Chlorhexidine and Cetrimide Steripods
Clorhexitulle
Colgen
Coltapaste
Corethium 1 and 2
Cuticerin
Cutifilm
Cutiplast
Debrisan Absorbent Pad
Dermalex
Dermasorb Spiral
Drawtex
Epiview
Fibracol
Fucidin Intertulle
Geliperm Dry Sheets and Granulate Gel
Granuflex hydrocolloid compression bandage
Histoacryl
Interface V–C
Jelonet (10 pieces)
Kaltocarb
Kaltoclude
Kaltogel
Kaltostat Fortex
Lyofoam A, K, Extra T and X

Malatex
Multidress
Multisorb
Neutratop Gel
Niko-Gard
Omiband
Ominatal
Opragel
Paratulle
Perfron
Pharmaclusive
Polybactrim
Poviderm
Rikospray
Serotulle
Sorbsan SA
Sofratulle
Spenco 2nd Skin
Spyrosorb
Sterigel
Sterijet Saline
Surfasoft
Tarband
Tegaderm Plus
Transite
Tribiotic
Variclene
Vigilon
Vivoderm

WOUND MANAGEMENT PRODUCTS IN THE DRUG TARIFF[260]

In the early 1980s, very few dressings were available apart from traditional dressings and paste bandages. The first representatives of modern wound management products became available in hospitals during the mid 1980s but did not become available in primary care until 1988 when Inadine, Granuflex, Kaltostat and Sorbsan were added to the Drug Tariff. Up until 1995, further products were cautiously added following careful evaluation. Many primary care practitioners e.g. nurses and wound care groups, complained about the limited choice in the Drug Tariff.

From 1996 (see **table**), however, this considered approach appears to have been abandoned as an avalanche of new products have been added both to the Drug Tariff and to the list of preparations which can be prescribed by nurses, Part XVIIB of the Drug Tariff. There is limited information available about these products e.g. evidence of effectiveness of individual products or of comparative effectiveness. In fact, when added to the Drug Tariff, it is often very difficult to find out basic details such as the name of the manufacturer of the product! Numbers of products added to the Drug Tariff each year were:

Year	Numbers	Year	Numbers
1988	4	1996	12
1989	1	1997	15
1990	4	1998	26
1991	4	1999	67
1992	2	2000	45
1993	5	2001	37
1994	4	2002	36
1995	5	2003	65
		2004 (until Sept)	40

CHARACTERISTICS OF IDEAL DRESSINGS[261]

1. Provide the optimum environment for wound healing – a moist environment – at the wound/dressing interface
2. Allow gaseous exchange of oxygen, carbon dioxide and water vapour
3. Provide thermal insulation – wound healing is temperature dependent
4. Impermeable to micro-organisms (in both directions)
5. Free from particulate contaminants
6. Non-adherent (many products are described as non-adherent but are low-adherent)
7. Safe to use (non-toxic, non-sensitising, non-allergenic)
8. Acceptable to the patient
9. High absorption characteristics (for exuding wounds)
10. Cost effective
11. Carrier for medicaments, e.g. antiseptics
12. Capable of standardisation and evaluation
13. Allow monitoring of the wound (transparent)
14. Provide mechanical protection
15. Non-inflammable
16. Sterilisable
17. Conformable and mouldable (especially over sacrum, heels and elbows)
18. Available (hospital and community) in a suitable range of forms and sizes
19. Require infrequent changing. Products should be left in place for as long as possible – "A bad cook always opens the oven door".

WOUND CARE GROUPS

American Academy of Wound Management Certifying board in the USA for healthcare professionals involved in wound care: www.aawm.org/

Association for the Advancement of Wound Care World-wide collaboration to advance the cause of wound care (based in the USA): www.AAWC1.com

Australian Wound Management Association www.awma.com.au/

British Lymphology Society BLS Administrative Centre, PO Box 1059, Caterham, Surrey CR3 6ZU. Tel: 01883 330253: www.lymphoedema.org

British Vascular Foundation Griffin House, West Street, Woking, Surrey GU21 1EB: www.bvf.org.uk

Cochrane Wounds Group 63 wound care reviews have been completed as of Issue 2 2004 (14 for pressure sores, 17 for venous ulcers and 13 for surgical wounds). These can be accessed at: www.cochrane.org or through the NHS Electronic Library www.nelh.nhs.uk

Community and District Nursing Association Thames Valley University, 8 University House, Ealing Green, London W5 5ED. Tel: 0208 2312776: www.cdna.tvu.ac.uk

European Pressure Ulcer Advisory Panel Wound Healing Unit, Department of Dermatology, Churchill Hospital, Old Road, Headington, Oxford OX3 7LJ. Fax: 01865 228233. www.epuap.org/

European Tissue Repair Society Aims to promote knowledge and improve contacts to those interested in the healing or related reactions of any organ. Secretariat: Department of Pathology, University of Geneva, 1 rue Michel Servet, 1211 Geneva 4, Switzerland. Tel: 0041 22 229 377: www.etrs.org/

European Wound Management Association Promotes advancement of education and research into native epidemiology, pathology, diagnosis, prevention and management of wounds of all aetiologies. Holds conferences and provides grants. PO Box 864, London SE1 8TT. Tel: 0207 848 3496: www.ewma.org/

Pressure Sore Web Forum An on-line discussion forum: www.medicaledu.com/forum.htm

The Leg Ulcer Forum CRICP, Wolfson Institute of Health Sciences, 32–38 Uxbridge Road, London W5 2BS. Tel: 0208 280 5020: www.legulcerforum.org

The Venous Forum Royal Society of Medicine, 1 Wimpole Street, London W1M 8AE. Tel: 0207 408 2119: www.rsm.ac.uk

Tissue Viability Nurses Association www.tvna.org

Tissue Viability Society Registered charity bringing together the multi-disciplinary skills of health care professionals in order to raise standards of good practice in the prevention and treatment of pressure sores, leg ulcers and chronic wounds. Glanville Centre, Salisbury District Hospital, Salisbury, Wilts SP2 8BJ. Tel: 01722 429057: www.tvs.org.uk/

Venous Stasis Ulcer Web Forum An on-line discussion forum www.medicaledu.com/venous_leg_ulcers

Wound Care Information Network www.medicaledu.com/

Wound Care Institute www.woundcare.org

Wound Care Society A charitable, non-profit based organisation whose main role is the provision of high quality wound care education. PO Box 170, Hartford, Huntingdon PE29 1PL. Tel/Fax: 01480 434401. www.woundcaresociety.org/

Wound Care Specialists multidisciplinary website dedicated to the interests of all wound care specialists: www.woundspecialist.com

Wound Care Web Forum medicaledu.com/wound_care_forum/

Wound Healing Society Non-profit, international organisation for those interested in the field of wound healing. www.woundhealsoc.org

Wound Ostomy Continence Nursing Society A professional nursing society which promotes educational, clinical, and research opportunities, to advance the practice and guide the delivery of expert healthcare to individuals with wounds, ostomies and incontinence. www.wocn.org/

World Union of Wound Healing Societies brings together all the major
scientific and sponsoring societies involved in wound care around the world.
www.wuwhs.org

WOUND CARE JOURNALS

Advances in Skin & Wound Care A scholarly, peer-reviewed,
multidisciplinary journal (formerly *Advances in Wound Care*) features original
research, comprehensive clinical reviews, and articles addressing practical
management of skin and wound care patients:
www.woundcarenet.com/advances.htm

Advances in Wound Care (*formerly Decubitus*) (Springhouse Corporation,
USA). Published bi-monthly

Journal of Tissue Viability (Tissue Viability Society, Salisbury). Published
quarterly: www.tvs.org.uk

Journal of Wound Care (emap Healthcare London). Published monthly:
www.journalofwoundcare.com/

Journal of Wound, Ostomy and Continence Nursing (Mosby, USA). An
authoritative resource devoted to the nursing care and management of patients
with abdominal stomas, wounds, pressure ulcers, fistulas, vascular ulcers and
incontinence: www1.mosby.com

Nursing Journal of the Tissue Viability Society Supplement in Nursing
Standard (RCN Publishing Company). Published quarterly

Ostomy/Wound Management Journal containing information on the care of
patients with ostomies, chronic wounds, incontinence, and related skin and
nutritional concerns: www.o-wm.com

Tissue Viability Supplement to British Journal of Nursing (Mark Allen
Publishing, London). Published quarterly: www.internurse.com

Wounds (Health Management Publications, USA). Published bi-monthly: www.woundsresearch.com/wnds/

Wound Repair and Regeneration The official publication of The Wound Healing Society, the European Tissue Repair Society, the Japanese Society for Wound Healing and the Australian Wound Management Association. Published six times a year. Contains original scientific and/or clinical papers on the broadly defined topics of wound healing and tissue regeneration: http://wizard.pharm.wayne.edu/wrr/WRR.HTM

World Wide Wounds Surgical Materials Testing Laboratory's electronic journal www.smtl.co.uk/World-Wide-Wounds/index.html

NURSE PRESCRIBERS' FORMULARY 2003–2005 (NPF)

The third edition of the NPF has been published. It succeeds earlier editions and two earlier pilot editions prepared for the nurse prescribing demonstration scheme. Subsequent editions will be published biennially. Information is set out as in the BNF and incorporates BNF 46 (Sept 2003). The NPF contains an extensive range of wound management dressings and related products including the following which may be prescribed by nurses on forms FP10P [FP10(N) in Scotland, form HS21(N) in Northern Ireland] for NHS patients:

- cavity dressings
- Chlorhexidine Gauze Dressing BP
- multi-layer compression bandaging
- silicone and silver -impregnated dressings
- soft polymer dressings
- zinc paste bandages (including both plain and with additional ingredients)

Framycetin Gauze Dressing BP and Sodium Fusidate Gauze Dressing BP are not on the Nurse Prescribers' Formulary.

A Prescribing Nurse Bulletin on dressings is available from the National Prescribing Centre website[262]: www.npc.co.uk

NICE GUIDELINES

All NICE appraisals and clinical guidelines are available from the NICE
website (www.nice.org.uk/).

Ref.	Guidance	Completed (not completed)	Review date
24	Use of debriding agents and specialist wound care clinics for difficult to heal surgical wounds	April 2001	Mar 2004
B	Pressure ulcer risk assessment and prevention (and a guide for patients and their carers)	April 2001	April 2005
CG7	Pressure ulcer risk assessment and prevention and equipment selection	Oct 2003	Oct 2007
CG10	Type 2 Diabetes. Prevention and management of foot problems	Jan 2004	Jan 2008
–	Pressure ulcer management	(August 2005)	
–	Surgical wounds, guidance on management	(April 2006)	
–	Woundcare suite including: Diabetic foot ulcers – new treatments Venous leg ulcers – new treatments	(to be confirmed)	

ADDITIONAL READING

1. Hollinworth H. Pain and wound care. Educational leaflet **7** (2). Hartford, Huntingdon: *The Wound Care Society*, 2000.
2. The World Union of Wound Healing Societies has produced its first international consensus document: Minimising pain at wound dressing - related procedures. The document is available from www.wuwhs.org as a downloadable pdf.
3. Culley F. Legal and professional issues in tissue viability revisited. Educational leaflet **7** (1). Hartford, Huntingdon: *The Wound Care Society*, 2000.
4. Collins F. Seating. Educational leaflet **8** (1). Hartford, Huntingdon: *The Wound Care Society*, 2001.
5. Lansdown A. Nutrition and the healing of skin wounds. Educational booklet **8** (2). Hartford, Huntingdon: *The Wound Care Society*, 2001.
6. Jackson L, Cutting K. Tissue Viability. Expert comment on key research papers selected from the international literature. Volume 1, part 3, December 2002. Current Medical Literature, London. (Available from your local Johnson & Johnson wound management representative.)
7. The European Wound Management Association have produced its third position statement on "Wound bed preparation in practice" – available from www.ewma.org as a downloadable pdf
8. Vowden K, Vowden P. Wound bed preparation. www.worldwidewounds.com/2002/april/Vowden/Wound-Bed-Preparation.html

WEB SITES – GENERAL

Biosurgical Research Unit (SMTL, Bridgend) Specialises in breeding maggots for sale and researching their use in wound care: www.larve.com

Dressing data cards SMTL have now launched data cards on a dedicated website: www.dressings.org/

Surgical Materials Testing Laboratory (Bridgend) Home page of SMTL, with links to World Wide Wounds and all related web sites. www.smtl.co.uk

SMTL Discussion Forum for wound management related issues www.smtl.co.uk/cgi-bin/HyperNews/get.cgi/wounds.html

MANUFACTURERS' WEB SITES

3M Healthcare	www.3mhealthcare.co.uk/
Beiersdorf Medical	www.beiersdorf-medical.com/
CliniMed	www.clinimed.co.uk
Coloplast	www.coloplast.co.uk
Coloplast newsletter (6-monthly)	www.woundmanagement.co.uk
ConvaTec	www.convatec.com/
Cook (for Oasis)	www.cookgroup.com
Hartmann	www.hartmann.co.uk
Kendall Healthcare	www.kendallhq.com
Mölnlycke	www.tendra.com
Smith & Nephew	www.smith-nephew.com
Vernon Carus	www.vernon-carus.co.uk

HELPLINES (freephones)

3M Health Care	0800 616066	
B Braun	0800 163007 (UK);	1800 409538 (Ireland)
CliniMed	0800 036900	
Coloplast	0800 220622 (UK);	1800 409502 (Ireland)
ConvaTec	0800 289738 (UK);	1800 721721 (Ireland)
Mölnlycke	0800 7311876	
S & N	0800 590173	
Unomedical	0800 214818	

OTHER HELPLINES

Robinson   01246 505450
Hartmann   01706 363290
Huntleigh   0345 585688 (Lo-call)

FINAL COMMENT – EMERGING DEVELOPMENTS

In the near future, there will be adjustments to the present range of products in the DT. A larger range of sizes and different shapes will become available e.g. shaped sacral and heel products. Many products will be available with and without borders, bevelled edges and adhesive. Some existing products may be deleted for wound care e.g. antiseptic and antibacterial products. There will be further developments to existing products e.g. use of silver-containing products and their mode of delivery.

New dressings will become available especially novel products for wounds which are difficult to heal. Collagen preparations have much potential as they are versatile and biocompatible. Regranex Gel is the first growth factor to be licensed for the treatment of diabetic ulcers. Progress, however, in using growth factors for wound care has been slow – when will other growth factors become available? Tissue-engineering will produce new products which substitute for skin or are equivalent to skin. Finally, gene therapy will emerge and it will be possible to treat wounds with healing genes.

Most of these new developments will be expensive and it will be interesting to observe their uptake by healthcare organisations. Cost effectiveness and the quality of the research data supporting the use of new products will be important determinants.

REFERENCES

1. Bradley M, Cullum N, Nelson EA, Petticrew M, Torgeson D. Systematic reviews of wound care management: (2) Dressings and topical agents used in the healing of chronic wounds. *Health Technol Assess* 1999; **3** (17 Pt 2).
2. Wounds: Venous leg ulcers. In Clinical Evidence. A compendium of the best available evidence for effective health care. BMJ Publishing Group, issue 2, Dec 1999.
3. Vermeulen H, Ubbink D, Goossens A, de Vos R, Legemate D. Dressings and topical agents for surgical wounds healing by secondary intention (Cochrane Review). In: The Cochrane Library, Issue 2, 2004, Chichester, UK: John Wiley & Sons, Ltd.
4. Falanga V, Williams R. The dark side of evidence-based wound management. *Journal of Wound Care* 2001;**10**(5): 145.
5. British National Formulary (current edition). British Medical Association and the Royal Pharmaceutical Society of Great Britain, London.
6. Vermeulen H, Ubbink D, Goossens A, de Vos R, Legemate D. Dressings and topical agents for surgical wounds healing by secondary intention (Cochrane Review). In: The Cochrane Library, Issue 2, 2004, Chichester, UK: John Wiley & Sons, Ltd).
7 Phillips I, Lobo AZ, Fernandes R, Gundara LS. Acetic acid in the treatment of superficial wounds infected by *Pseudomonas aeruginosa*. *Lancet* 1968; **1:** 11–13
8. Milner SM. Acetic acid to treat *Pseudomonas aeruginosa* in superficial wounds and burns. *Lancet* 1992; **340:** 61 (letter)
9. Charters A. Wound glue: a comparative study of tissue adhesives. *Accident and Emergency Nursing* 2000; **8:** 223–227.
10. Farion K, Osmond MH, Hartling L, Russell K, Klassen T, Crumley E, Wiebe N. Tissue adhesives for traumatic lacerations in children and adults (Cochrane Review). In: The Cochrane Library, Issue 3. Oxford: Update Software, 2002
11. Coulthard P, Worthington H, Esposito M, van der Elst M, van Waes OJF. Tissue adhesives for the closure of surgical incisions. (Cochrane Review) In: The Cochrane Library, Issue 2, 2004, Chichester, UK: John Wiley & Sons, Ltd
12. Application of alcohol (reader's question). *J Wound Care* 1992; **1**(2):53
13. Morgan DA. Alginate dressings. Part 1: Historical Aspects. *J Tissue Viability* 1997; **7**(1): 4–9
14 Morgan DA. Alginate dressings. Part 2: Product Guide. *J Tissue Viability* 1997; **7**(1): 9–14.
15. Thomas S, Loveless P. Observations on the fluid handling properties of alginate dressings. *Pharm J* 1992; **248:** 850–851
16. Johnson BJ, Simpson C. A laboratory comparison of alginate dressings. *Pharm J* 1993. **251:** 46
17. Agren MS. Four alginate dressings in the treatment of partial thickness wounds: a comparative experimental study. *Br J Plastic Surgery* 1996; **49**(2): 129–134.
18. Berry DP, Bale S, Harding KG. Dressings for treating cavity wounds. *J Wound Care* 1996; **5**(1): 10–13
19. Sayag J, Meaume S, Bohbot S. Healing properties of calcium alginate dressings. *J Wound Care* 1996; **5**(8): 357–362
20. Bale S, Squires D, Varnon T, Walker A, Benbow M, Harding KG. A comparison of two dressings in pressure sore management. *J Wound Care* 1997; **6**(10): 463–466.
21. Butterworth RJ, *et al.* Comparing Allevyn Cavity Wound Dressings and Silastic Foam. *J Wound Care* 1992 ; **1**(1) : 10–13.
22. Infection control in general practice Part 5: topical drugs. *Supplement to MIMS Magazine* 1993; 29 June: 1–8
23. Lineaweaver W, Howard R, Soucy D et al. Topical Antimicrobial toxicity. *Arch Surg* 1985; **120:** 267–270
24 Morison M. Wound Cleansing—Which Solution? *Nursing Standard* 1990; **4**(52): 4–6
25. Liptak JM. An overview of the topical management of wounds. *Austral Vet* 1997; **75**(6): 408–413.

26. Leaper DJ, Simpson RA. The effect of antiseptics and topical antimicrobials on wound healing. *J Antimicrob Chemother* 1986; **17:** 135–137
27. Morgan DA. Is there still a role for antiseptics? *J Tissue Viability* 1993; **3**(3): 80–84
28. Lawrence JC, Harding KG, Moore DJ. The use of antiseptics in wound care. *J Wound Care* 1996; **5**(1): 44–47
29. Mimoz O, Karim A, Mercat A *et al.* Chlorhexidine compared with povidone-iodine as skin preparation before blood culture. *Ann Intern Med.* 1999; **131:** 834–837
30. Scanlon E. To use or not to use? The debate on the use of antiseptics in wound care. *WoundCare* 2002: September: 8–20.
31. Cooper R. A review of the evidence for the use of topical antimicrobial agents in wound care. www.worldwidewounds.com/2004/february/cooper/Topical-Antimicrobial-Agents.html
32. Armstrong SH, Ruckley CV. Use of a fibrous dressing in exuding leg ulcers. *J Wound Care* 1997; **6**(7): 322–324
33. Thomas S, Hay NP. *In vitro* investigations of a new hydrogel dressing. *J Wound Care* 1996; **5**(3): 130–131
34. Layton AM, Ibbotson SH, Davies JA, Goodfield MJD. Randomised trial of oral aspirin for chronic venous leg ulcers. *Lancet* 1994; **344:** 164–165
35. Ibbotson SH *et al.* The effect of aspirin on haemostatic activity in the treatment of chronic venous leg ulceration. *Br J Dermatol* 1995; **132:** 422–426
36. Ruckley CV, Prescott RA. Treatment of chronic leg ulcers. *Lancet* 1994; **344:** 1512–1513
37. Thomas S *et al.* Improvements in medicated tulle dressings. *J Hosp Infect* 1983; **4:** 391–398
38. British Standards Institution. British Standard 7505: elastic properties of flat, non-adhesive, extensible fabric bandages. Milton Keynes: BSI, 1995
39. Thomas S, Toyick N, Fisher B. Graduated external compression and the prevention of deep vein thrombosis. Surgical Materials Testing Laboratory, Bridgend 2000
40. Lawrence JC. A first-aid preparation for burns and scalds. *J Wound Care* 1996; **5:** 262–4
41. Dunn RJ. Practical application of a first-aid treatment for burns and scalds. *J Wound Care* 1996; **5:** 265–6
42. Rotheli-Simmen B, Martinelli E, Muhlebach S. Formulation of a stable calcium gluconate gel for topical treatment of hydrofluoric acid burns. *EHP* 1996; **2:** 176–80
43. Wood RAB. Foam elastomer dressing in the management of open granulating wounds: experience with 280 patients. *Br J Surg* 1977; **64:** 554–7
44. Cooper R, Bale S, Harding JG. An improved cleaning regime for a modified foam cavity dressing. *J Wound Care* 1995; **4:** 13–6
45. Thomas S, Hay N.P, Wound Cleansing. *Pharm J* 1985; **235:** 206 (letter)
46. McLure AR, Gordon J. *In vitro* evaluation of povidone-iodine and chlorhexidine against methicillin-resistant Staphylococcus aureus. *J Hosp Infect* 1992; **21:** 291–9
47. Cheung J, O'Leary JJ. Allergic reaction to chlorhexidine in an anaesthetised patient. *Anaesth Intensive Care* 1985; **13:** 429–30
48. Evans RJ. Acute anaphylaxis due to topical chlorhexidine acetate. *Br Med J* 1992; **304:** 686 (letter)
49. Drosou A, Falabella A, Kirsner RS. Antiseptics on wounds: an area of controversy. *Wounds* 2003; **15**(5): 149–66
50. Morgan DA. Wound Care: Chlorinated Solutions—E(useful) or (e)useless. *Pharm J* 1989; **243:** 219–20
51. Morgan DA. Chlorinated Solutions—An Update. *J Tissue Viability* 1991; **1:** 31–3
52. Moore D. Hypochlorites : a review of the evidence. *J Wound Care* 1992 ; **1:** 44 - 53
53. Tatnall FM, Leigh IM, Gibson JR. Comparative study of antiseptic toxicity on basal keratinocytes, transformed human keratinocytes and fibroblasts. *Skin Pharmacol* 1990; **3:** 157–63
54. Cannavo M, Fairbrother G, Owen D, Ingle J, Lumley T. J *Wound Care* 1998; **7:** 57–62
55. Burgess B. An investigation of hydrocolloids. A comparative prospective randomised trial of the performance of three hydrocolloid dressings. *Professional Nurse Supplement* 1993; **8:** 3–6

56. Stockport JC, Groarke L, Ellison DA, McCollum C. Single-layer and multilayer bandaging in the treatment of venous leg ulcers. *J Wound Care* 1997; **6**(10): 485–488
57. Thomas S, Fram P. An evaluation of a new type of compression bandaging system. www.worldwidewounds.com/2003/september
58. Morrell CJ, Walters SJ, Dixon S *et al.* Cost effectiveness of community leg ulcer clinics: randomised controlled trial. *Br Med J* 1998; **316**: 1487–1491
59. Cullum N, Nelson EA, Fletcher AW, Sheldon TA, Song F, Fletcher AW. Compression for venous leg ulcers (Cochrane Review). In: *Cochrane Library*, Issue 3, 2000. Oxford: Update Software
60. Compression therapy for venous leg ulcers. *Effective Health Care Bulletin* 1997; **3**: 1-12
61. Carr L, Phillips Z, Posnett J. Comparative cost-effectiveness of four layer bandaging in the treatment of venous leg ulceration. *J Wound Care* 1999; **8**: 243–248
62. Moffatt CJ, Dickson D. The Charing Cross high compression four-layer bandage system. *J Wound Care* 1993; **2**(2): 91–94
63. Johnson S. Compression hosiery in the prevention and treatment of venous leg ulcers. *J Tissue Viability* 2002; **12**: 67–74
64. Young G. Compression hosiery: guide to types and recommended use. *Prescriber* 2004; **15**(2): 34–39
65. Bennett G. Graduated compression hosiery. Educational leaflet 6 (1). Hartford, Huntingdon: *The Wound Care Society*, 1999.
66. Agu O, Hamilton G, Baker D. Graduated compression stockings in the prevention of venous thromboembolism. *British Journal of Surgery* 1999; **86**: 992–1004
67. Amaragiri SV, Lees TA. Elastic compression stockings for prevention of deep vein thrombosis (Cochrane Review). In: The Cochrane Library, Issue 2, 2004, Chichester, UK: John Wiley & Sons, Ltd
68. Glyantsev SP, Adamyan AA, Sakharov IYu. Crab collagenase in wound debridement. *J Wound Care* 1997; **6**(1): 13–16
69. Thomas S, Fear M. Comparing two dressings for wound debridement. *J Wound Care* 1993; **2**(5): 272–274
70. Colin D, Kurring PA, Quinlan D, Yvon C. Managing sloughy pressure sores. *J Wound Care* 1996; **5**(10): 444–446
71. Thomas S, Fisher B, Fram PJ, Waring MJ. Odour-absorbing dressings. *J Wound Care* 1998; **7**(5): 246–250
72. Bowler PG, Davies BJ, Jones SA. Microbial involvement in chronic wound malodour. *J Wound Care* 1999; **8**: 216–218
73. Morgan DA. *Wound Cleansing Agents.* Educational Leaflet No. 10 (Parts 1 and 2). The Wound Care Society 1992
74. Bradley M, Cullum N, Sheldon T. The debridement of chronic wounds: a systematic review. *Health Technol Assess* 1999; **3** (17 Pt 1)
75. Thomas S. Opinion: NICE – time for review? *World Wide Wounds* June 2001, www.smtl.co.uk/
76. Hallett A. Hampton S. Wound dressings. Educational leaflet 6 (1). Hartford, Huntingdon: *The Wound Care Society,* 1999.
77. Thomas S. The importance of secondary dressings in wound care. *J Wound Care* 1998; **7**(4): 189–192
78. Staunton NA. Novel approach to the supply of dressings. *Prescriber* 2002; **13**(16): 19-21
79. Hallworth R. Wound management starter pack initiative. *Prescriber* 2003; 19 June: 14-21
80. Bowler *et al.* The viral barrier properties of some occlusive dressings and their control in infection control. *Wounds* 1993; **5**(1): 1–8
81. Salmonella and raw eggs. Executive Letter DoH, 5 Sept. 1988. EL (88) CO/10
82. Baker J. Essential oils: a complementary therapy in wound management. *J Wound Care* 1998; **7**(7): 355–357
83. Leaper DJ. Eusol (Editorial). *Br Med J* 1992; **304**: 930–931

84. Payne CMER et al. Argyria from excessive use of topical silver sulphadiazine. *Lancet* 1992; **340:** 126 (letter)

85. Bugmann Ph, Taylor S, Gyger D et al. A silicone-coated nylon dressing reduces healing time in burned paediatric patients in comparison with standard sulfadiazine treatment: a prospective randomised trial. *Burns* 1998; **24:** 609–612

86. Thomas S, Loveless P. Examining the properties and uses of two hydrogel sheet dressings. *J Wound Care* 1993; **2**(3): 176–179

87. Thomas S, Banks V, Bale S, Fear-Price M, Hagelstein S, Harding KG, Orpin J, Thomas N. A comparison of two dressings in the management of chronic wounds. *J Wound Care* 1997; **6**(8): 383–386

88. Harding K, Cutting KF, Price P. The cost-effectiveness of wound management protocols of care. *British Journal of Nursing* 2000 (supplement); **9** (19): S6–S24

89. Young SR, Dyson M, Hickman R, Lang S, Osborn C. Comparison of the effects of semi-occlusive polyurethane dressings and hydrocolloid dressings on dermal repair: 1. Cellular changes. *J Invest Dermatol* 1991; **97:** 586–592

90. Phillips TJ, Palko MJ, Bhawan J. Histologic evaluation of chronic human wounds treated with hydrocolloid and non-hydrocolloid dressings. *J Am Acad Dermatol* 1994; **30:** 61–64

91. Glover M. Growth Factors and Wound Healing. *Wound Management* 1992; **2**(1): 9–11

92. Hopkinson I. Growth Factors and extracellular matrix biosynthesis. *J Wound Care* 1992; **1**(2): 47–50

93. Falanga V. Growth Factors and Wound Repair. *J Tissue Viability* 1992; **2**(3): 101–104

94. Arnold F, O'Brien J, Cherry G. Granulocyte monocyte-colony stimulating factor as an agent for wound healing. *J Wound Care* 1995; **4**(9): 400–402

95. Singer AJ, Clark RAF. Cutaneous wound healing. *New Engl J Med* 1999; **341**(10): 738–746

96. Garrett B, Garrett SB. Cellular communication and the action of growth factors during wound healing. *J Wound Care* 1997; **6**(6): 277–280

97. Carter K. Growth factors: the wound healing therapy of the future? *WoundCare* 2003; September: S15–S23

98. Zumla A, Lulet A. Honey—a remedy rediscovered. *J Roy Soc Med* 1989; **82:** 384–385

99. Molan PC. Honey as a topical antibacterial agent for treatment of infected wounds. www.worldwidewounds.com/2001/november/Molan

100. Cooper R. A review of the evidence for the use of topical antimicrobial agents in wound care. www.worldwidewounds.com/2004/february/Cooper/Topical-Antimicrobial-Agents

101. Willix DJ, Molan PC, Harfoot CG. A comparison of the sensitivity of wound-infecting species of bacteria to the antibacterial activity of manuka honey and other honey. *J Appl Bact* 1992; **73:** 388–394

102. Molan PC. A brief review of honey as a clinical dressing. *Primary Intention* 1998; **6**(4): 148–158

103. Molan PC. The role of honey in the management of wounds. *J Wound Care* 1999; **8**(8): 415–418

104. Subrahmanyam M. A prospective clinical and histological study of superficial burn wound healing with honey and silver sulfadiazine. *Burns* 1998; **24**(2): 157–161

105. Cooper R, Molan PC. The use of honey as an antiseptic in managing Pseudomonas infection. *J Wound Care* 1999; **8**(4): 161–164

106. Cooper RA, Molan PC. Honey in wound care. *J Wound Care* 1999; **8**(7): 340

107. Postmes T, Van Den Bogaard AE, Hazen M. Honey for wounds, ulcers and skin graft preservation. *Lancet* 1993; **341:** 756–757 (letter)

108. Cooper RA, Molan PC, Harding KG. The sensitivity to honey of gram-positive cocci of clinical significance isolated from wounds. *J of Applied Microbiology* 2002; **93:** 857–863

109. Margolis DJ, Knauss J, Bilkor W. Hormone replacement therapy and prevention of pressure ulcers and venous leg ulcers. *Lancet* 2002; **359:** 675–677

110. Rousseau P, Niecestro RM. Comparison of the physicochemical properties of various hydrocolloid dressings. *Wounds* 1991; **3**(1): 43–48

111. Thomas S, Loveless P. A comparative study of the properties of six hydrocolloid dressings. *Pharm J* 1991; **247:** 672–675

112. Hutchinson JJ. A prospective clinical trial of wound dressings to investigate the rate of infection under occlusion. In: Proceedings of the 3rd European Conference on Advances in Wound Management, eds, Harding KG, Dealey C, Cherry & Finn Gottrup, 1994; 93–96. London: Macmillan Magazines

113. Hutchinson JJ, Lawrence JC. Wound infection under occlusive dressings. *J Hosp Infect* 1991; **17:** 83–94

114. Gill D. The use of hydrocolloids in the treatment of diabetic foot. *J Wound Care* 1999; **8**(4): 204–206

115. Agren M. The cytocompatibility of hydrocolloid dressings. *J Wound Care* 1997; **6**(6): 272–274

116. Sleigh JW, Linter SPK. Hazards of hydrogen peroxide. *Br Med J* 1985; **291:** 1706

117. *Journal of the Medical Defence Union* (Winter, 1988)

118. Simon RH, Scoggin CH, Patterson D. Hydrogen peroxide causes the fatal injury to human fibroblasts exposed to oxygen radicals. *J Biological Chemistry* 1981; **256:** 7181–7186

119. Schmidt RJ, Chung LY, Andrews AM, Turner TD. Hydrogen peroxide is a murine (L929) fibroblast cell proliferant at micro- to manomolar concentrations. In: Proceedings of 1st European Conference on Advances in Wound Management, eds Harding KG, Leaper DL, Turner TD 1992: 117–120. London: Macmillan

120. McKenna PJ, Lehr GS, Leist P, Welling RE. Antiseptic effectiveness with fibroblast preservation. *Annals of Plastic Surgery* 1991; **27:** 265–268

121. Cooper R. A review of the evidence for the use of topical antimicrobial agents in wound care. www.worldwidewounds.com/2004/february/Cooper/Topical-Antimicrobial-Agents

122. Greenway SE. Filler LE. Greenway FL. Topical insulin in wound healing: a randomised, double-blind, placebo-controlled trial. *J Wound Care* 1999; **8**(10): 526–528

123. Bale S, Banks V, Harding KG. A comparison of two amorphous hydrogels in the debridement of pressure sores. *J Wound Care* 1998; **7**(2): 65–68

124. Thomas S. Assessing the hydro-affinity of hydrogel dressings. *J Wound Care* 1994; **3**(2): 89–91

125. Gilchrist B. Should iodine be reconsidered in wound management. *J Wound Care* 1997; **6** (3): 148–150

126. Kero M *et al.* A comparison of Cadexomer Iodine with Dextranomer in the treatment of venous leg ulcers. *Curr Therap Res* 1987 (Nov); **42**(5): 761–767

127. Williams P *et al.* A comparison of two alginate dressings in the management of acute wound cavities. In: Proceedings of the 4th European Conference on Advances in Wound Management, eds Cherry GW, Leaper DJ, Lawrence JC, Milward P, 1995; 55–56. London, Macmillan Magazines

128. Martin SJ, Corrado OJ, Kay EA. Enzymatic debridement for necrotic wounds. *J Wound Care* 1996; **5**(7): 310–311

129. Thomas S. Advice for community pharmacists on how to order and dispose of maggots. *The Pharmaceutical Journal* 2004; **272:** 222–3

130. Thomas S, Andrews A, Hay P, Bourgoise S. The anti-microbial activity of maggot secretions: results of a preliminary study. *J Tissue Viability* 1999; **9**(6): 127–132)

131. Thomas S, Jones M. Maggots and the battle against MRSA: an ancient solution to a modern problem. Biosurgical Research Unit, Bridgend 2000

132. Thomas S, Andrews A, Jones M. The use of larval therapy in wound management. *J Wound Care* 1998; **7**(10): 521–524

133. Courtenay M. The use of larval therapy in wound management in the UK. *J Wound Care* 1999; **8**(4): 177–179

134. Thomas S, McCubbin P. Use of maggots in the care of wounds. *Hospital Pharmacist* 2002; **9:** 267–271

135. Wayman J, Nirojogi V, Walker A, Sowinski A, Walker MA. The cost effectiveness of larval therapy in venous ulcers. *J Tissue Viability* 2000; **10**(3): 91–94

136. Charters A. Wound glue: a comparative study of tissue adhesives. *Accident and Emergency Nursing* 2000; **8:** 223–227

137. Hinshaw J. Larval therapy: a review of clinical human and veterinary studies. *World Wide Wounds* October 2000 (www.worldwidewounds.com/2000/oct/Janet-Hinshaw/Larval-Therapy-Human-and-Veterinary.html)

138. Morgan DA. Myiasis: The rise and fall of maggot therapy. *J Tissue Viability* 1995; **5**(2): 43–51

139. Thomas S, Jones M, Shutler S, Jones S. Using larvae in modern wound management. *J Wound Care* 1996; **5**(2): 60–69

140. Thomas S, Andrews A. The effect of hydrogel dressings on maggot development. *J Wound Care* 1999; **8**: 75–77

141. Bugmann Ph, Taylor S, Gyger D *et al*. A silicone-coated nylon dressing reduces healing time in burned paediatric patients in comparison with standard sulfadiazine treatment: a prospective randomised trial. *Burns* 1998; **24:** 609–612

142. Editorial. Management of Smelly Tumours. *Lancet* 1990; **355:** 141–142

143. Thompson Rice J. Metronidazole use in malodorous skin lesions. *Rehabilitation Nursing* 1992; **17**(5): 244–245, 255

144. Metronidazole gel for smelly tumours. *Drug Ther Bulletin* 1992; **30:** 18–9

145. Hampson JP. The use of metronidazole in the treatment of malodorous wounds. *J Wound Care* 1996; **5**(9): 421–426

146. Witte MB, Kiyama T, Barbul A. Nitric oxide enhances experimental wound healing in diabetes. *Br J Surg* 2002; **89:** 1594–1601

147. Lawrence JC, Kidson A, Lilly HA. An adherent semi-permeable film dressing for burns. *J Wound Care* 1992; **1**(2): 10–11

148. Anonymous. Paroven: not much effect in trials (review). *Drug Therap Bull* 1992; **30**(2): 7–8

149. Heng MC, Pilgrim JP, Beck FW. A simplified hyperbaric oxygen technique for leg ulcers (clinical trial). *Arch Derm* 1984; **120**(5): 640–645

150. Greif R, Akca O, Horn E-P, Kurz A, Sessler DI. Supplemental perioperative oxygen to reduce the incidence of surgical-wound infection. *N Engl J Med* 2000; **342:** 161–167

151. Cutting K. Hyperbaric oxygen therapy. *NTPlus* 2001; **97**(9): VII

152. Kranke P, Bennett M, Roeckl-Wiedmann I, Debus S. Hyperbaric oxygen therapy for chronic wounds. (Cochrane Review) In: The Cochrane Library, Issue 2, 2004, Chichester, UK: John Wiley & Sons, Ltd

153. Powell SM *et al*. Patch test study of a new medicated paste bandage in patients with chronic leg ulcers. In: Proceedings of the 4th European Conference on Advances in Wound Management, eds, Cherry GW, Leaper DJ, Lawrence JC, Milward P. 1995; 66–68. London, Macmillan Magazines

154. Stacey MC, Jopp-Mckay AG, Rashid P, Hoskin SE, Thompson PJ. The influence of dressings on venous ulcer healing – a randomised trial. *Eur J Vasc Endovasc Surg* 1997; **13:** 174–179

155. Oxpentifylline for venous leg ulcers. *Drug Therap Bull* 1991; **29:** 59–60

156. Jull AB, Waters J, Arrol B. Oral pentoxifylline for treatment of venous leg ulcers (Cochrane Review). In: *Cochrane Library*, Issue 3, 2000. Oxford: Update Software

157. Dale JJ, Ruckley CV, Harper DR, Gibson B, Nelson EA, Prescott RJ. Randomised, double blind placebo controlled trial of pentoxifylline in the treatment of venous leg ulcers. *Br Med J* 1999; **319:** 875–878

158. Belcaro G, Cesarone MR, Nicolaides AN et al. Treatment of venous ulcers with Pentoxifylline: a 6-month randomized double-blind, placebo controlled trial. *Angiology* 2002; **53** (suppl 1): S45–S47

159. De Sanctis MT, Belcaro G, Cesarone MR et al. Treatment of venous ulcers with Pentoxifylline: a 12-month double-blind, placebo controlled trial. Microcirculation and healing. *Angiology* 2002; **53** (suppl 1): S49–S51

160. Jull AB, Waters J, Arroll B. Pentoxifylline for treating venous leg ulcers (Cochrane Review). In: The Cochrane Library, Issue 2, 2004. Chichester, UK: John Wiley & Sons, Ltd

161. Anstead GM, Hart LM, Sunahara JF, Liter ME. Phenytoin in wound healing. *Ann Pharmacother* 1996; **30:** 768–775

162. Lodha SC *et al*. Role of phenytoin in healing of large abscess cavities. *Br J Surg* 1991; **78:**

105–108
163. Rhodes RS *et al.* Topical phenytoin treatment of stage II decubitus ulcers in the elderly. *Ann Pharmacother* 2001; **35:** 675–81
164. Simon DA, Dix FP, McCollum CN. Management of venous leg ulcers. *BMJ* 2004; **328:** 1358–1362
165. Gilmore OJA, Reid C, Strokon A. A study of the effect of povidone-iodine on wound healing. *Postgrad Med J* 1977; **53:** 617, 122–125
166. Waran KD, Munsick RA. Anaphylaxis from povidone-iodine. *Lancet* 1995; **345:** 1506
167. Flynn J. Povidone-iodine as a topical antiseptic for treating and preventing wound infection: a literature review. *WoundCare* 2003; June: 36–42
168. Fenton AH, Warren M. Release of medicament from proflavine cream. *Pharm J* 1962; **188:** 5
169. Gupta R, Foster ME, Miller E. Calcium alginate in the management of acute surgical wounds and abscesses. *J Tissue Viability* 1991; **1**(4): 115–116
170. Moore PJ, Foster L. Managing surgical wounds: two dressings reviewed. *British Journal of Health Care Management* 2001; **7** (2): 75–77
171. Ghatnekar O, Persson U, Willis M, Odegaard K. Cost effectiveness of becaplermin in the treatment of diabetic foot ulcers in four European countries. *Pharmocoeconomics* 2001; **19**(7): 767–778
172. Sawada Y, Sone K. Treatment of scars and keloids with a cream containing silicone oil. *Br J Plast Surg* 1990; **43:** 683–688
173. Sawada Y, Sone K. Beneficial effects of silicone cream on grafted skin. *Br J Plast Surg* 1992; **45:** 105–108
174. Mustoe TA. Cooter RD, Gold MH, Hobbs FDR, et al. International clinical recommendations on scar management. *Plast Reconstr Surg* 2002; **110**(2): 560–71
175. Lansdown ABG. Silver in wound care and management. Educational leaflet 3 (1). Hartford, Huntingdon: *The Wound Care Society,* 2003.
176. Thurman RB, Gerba CP. The molecular mechanisms of copper and silver ion disinfection of bacteria and viruses. *CRC Critical Reviews in Environmental Control* 1989; **18**(4): 295-315
177. Thomas S, McCubbin P. A comparison of the antimicrobial effects of four silver-containing dressings on three organisms. *J Wound Care* 2003; **12:** 101–107
178. Dealey C. Using protective skin wipes under adhesive tapes. *J Wound Care* 1992; **1:** 19–22
179. Mulder GT. The role of tissue engineering in wound care. *J Wound Care* 1999; **8**(1): 21–24.
180. A code of practice for the production of human-derived therapeutic products. Medical Devices Agency, July 2002
181. Wong LS, Green HM, Feugate JE, Yadav M, Nothnagel EA, Martins-Green M. Effects of "second-hand" smoke on structure and function of fibroblasts, cells that are critical for tissue repair and remodeling. *BMC Cell Biology* 2004; **5:** 13
182. Whiteford L. Nicotine, CO and HCN: the detrimental effects of smoking on wound healing. *WoundCare,* December 2003, S22–S26
183. Ernst AA, Gershoff L, Miller P, Tilden E, Weiss SJ. Warmed versus room temperature saline for laceration irrigation: a randomized clinical trial. *Southern Med J* 2003; **96:** 436–60
184. Anon. Spray-on biodegradable fibres to help heal wounds. *Pharm J* 2000; **264:** 87
185. Tsakayannis D *et al.* Sucralfate and chronic venous stasis ulcers. *Lancet* 1994; **343:** 424–425
186. Topham J. Sugar for wounds. *J Tissue Viability* 2000; **10**(3): 86–89
187. Middleton KR, Seal D. Sugar as an aid to wound healing. *Pharm J* 1985; **235:** 757–758
188. Archer *et al.* A controlled model of moist wound healing: comparison between semi-permeable film, antiseptics and sugar paste. *J Exp Path* 1990; **71:** 155–170
189. Ambrose U, Middleton K, Seal D. *In Vitro* studies of water activity and bacterial growth inhibition of sucrose-polyethylene glycol 400-hydrogen peroxide and xylose-polyethylene glycol 400-hydrogen peroxide pastes used to treat infected wounds. *Antimicrob Agents Chemother* 1991; **35**(9): 1799–1803
190. Anon. Cleansing wounds with tap water. *J Wound Care* 1994; **3**(2): 65
191. Angeras AD *et al.* Comparison between sterile saline and tap water for the cleansing of acute traumatic soft tissue wounds. *Eur J Surg* 1992; **158**(33): 347–350

192. Riyat MS, Quinton DN. Tap water as a wound cleansing agent in accident and emergency. *J Acc Emerg Med* 1997; **14:** 165–166

193. Valente JH, Forti RJ, Freundlich LF, Zandieh SO, Crain EF. Wound irrigation in children: saline solution or tap water? *Ann Emerg Med* 2003; **41:** 609–16

194. Fernandez R, Griffiths R, Ussia C. Water for wound cleansing (Cochrane Review). In: The Cochrane Library, Issue 2, 2004, Chichester, UK: John Wiley & Sons, Ltd

195. Lawrence JC. Medicated tulle dressings. *J Wound Care* 1993; **2**(4): 240–243

196. Deeth M. Review of an independent audit into the clinical efficacy of Vacutex. *Br J Nursing* 2002 (supplement); **11**(12): S60–66

197. Baxandall T. Healing cavity wounds with negative pressure. *Nursing Standard* 1996; **11**(6): 49–51

198. Ballard K, Baxter H. Vacuum-assisted closure. *NTPlus* 2001; **97**(35): 51-52

199. Thomas S. Vapour-permeable film dressings. *J Wound Care* 1996; **5**(6): 271–274

200. Thomas S, Loveless P, Hay NP. Comparative review of the properties of six semi-permeable film dressings. *Pharm J* 1988; **240:** 785–789

201. Hoffmann *et al*. Transparent polyurethane film as an intravenous catheter dressing. A meta-analysis of the infection risks. *JAMA* 1992; **267**(15): 2072–2076

202. Gillies D, O'Riordan L, Carr D, Gunning R, O'Brien I. Gauze and tape and transparent polyurethane dressings for central venous catheters (Cochrane Methodology Review). In: The Cochrane Library, Issue 4, 2003. Chichester, UK: John Wiley & Sons, Ltd

203. McKeeman K, Wallace P. Bring Varidase use into line. A drug use evaluation of Varidase Topical solution. *Pharmacy in Practice* 1995; September: 336–339

204. Green C. Antistreptokinase titres after topical streptokinase. *Lancet* 1993; **341:** 1602–1603

205. Bux M, Baig MK, Rodrigues E, Armstrong D, Brown A. Antibody response to topical streptokinase *J Wound Care* 1997; **6**(2): 70–73

206. Wilkinson EAJ, Hawke CI. Does oral zinc aid the healing of chronic leg ulcers? (Cochrane Review). In: *The Cochrane Library*, Issue 4, 1998. Oxford: Update Software

207. Morgan DA. Wounds – what should a dressings formulary include? *Hospital Pharmacist* 2002; **9:** 261–266

208. Guidelines for wound management in Northern Ireland. Clinical Resource Efficiency Support Team. October 1998, Belfast

209. Vowden K. Vowden P. Leg ulcer assessment. Educational leaflet 5 (3). Hartford, Huntingdon: *The Wound Care Society,* 1998.

210. Tong A. The Principles of Assessment and Management of Burn Injuries. Educational booklet 8 (4). Hartford, Huntingdon: *The Wound Care Society,* 2002.

211. Hettiaratchy S, Dziewulski P. ABC of burns: an introduction. *BMJ* 2004; **328:** 1366–1368

212. Berry DP, Jones V. Cavity wound management. *J Wound Care* 1993; **2**(1): 29–32

213. Bale S. Cavity wounds. Educational leaflet No. 11. *The Wound Care Society* 1993

214. Swartz MN. Cellulitis. *NEJM* 2004; **350:** 904–912

215. Complications of diabetes: screening for retinopathy, management of foot ulcers. *Effective Health Care August* 1999; **5**(4). The University of York. NHS Centre for Reviews and Dissemination

216. Spencer S. Pressure relieving interventions for preventing and treating diabetic foot ulcers (Cochrane Review). In: *Cochrane Library*, Issue 3, 2000. Oxford: Update Software

217. The Diabetic Foot. Educational leaflet 7 (4). Hartford, Huntingdon: *The Wound Care Society,* 2000.

218. Jeffcoate WJ, Harding KG. Diabetic foot ulcers. *Lancet* 2003; **361:** 1545–51

219. Clinical guideline 10. Type 2 Diabetes. Prevention and management of foot problems. NICE January 2004.

220. Managing foot ulcers in patients with diabetes. *DTB* 2002; **40:** 11-14. Consumers Association, London.

221. Clinical guideline 10. Type 2 Diabetes. Prevention and management of foot problems. *NICE* January 2004

222. Andrew JM, Boulton MD, Robert S, Kirsner MD, Vileikyte MD. Neuropathic diabetic foot ulcers. *New England Journal of Medicine* 2004; **351:** 48–55

223. Beldon P. Skin grafts 2: management of donor site wounds in the community. *WoundCare* September 2003: S6–S14
224. White RJ. The management of exuding wounds. Educational leaflet 7 (3). Hartford, Huntingdon: *The Wound Care Society*, 2000.
225. White R. Managing exudate (part 1). *NTPlus* 2001; **97** (9): XI–XIII
226. White R. Managing exudate (part 2). *NTPlus* 2001; **97** (14): 59–60
227. Cutting KF. Wounds and infection. Educational leaflet 5 (2). Hartford, Huntingdon: *The Wound Care Society,* 1998.
228. Kingsley A. A proactive approach to wound infection. *Nurs Stand* 2001; **15**(30): 50–58
229. Cutting KF, White R. Defined and redefined: criteria for identifying wound infection revisited. *WoundCare* 2004; March: S6–15
230. Collier M. Recognition and management of wound infections. www.worldwidewounds com/2004/january/Collier
231. Naylor W. Part 1: Symptom control in the management of fungating wounds. www.worldwidewounds.com/2002/march/Naylor/Symptom-Control-Fungating-Wounds.html
232. Grocott P. Palliative management of fungating malignant wounds. Educational booklet 8 (2). Hartford, Huntingdon: *The Wound Care Society*, 2001.
233. Leaper D. Sharp technique for wound debridement. www.worldwidewounds.com/2002/december.
234. O'Brien M. Exploring methods of wound debridement. *WoundCare* 2002; December: 10–18
235. NICE Technology Appraisal Guidance No 24 – Guidance on the use of debriding agents and specialist wound care clinics for difficult to heal surgical wounds (April 2001)
236. Vowden K. The use of intermittent pneumatic compression in venous ulceration. *British Journal of Nursing* 2001; **10**(8): 491–509
237. Dunford C. Hypergranulation tissue. *J Wound Care* 1999; **8**: 506–7
238. Harris A, Rolstad BS. Hypergranulation tissue: a non-traumatic method of management. In: Proceedings of the 2nd European Conference on Advances in Wound Management, Harding KG, Cherry G, Dealey C, Turner TD, editors. London, Macmillan Magazines Ltd, 1993: 35–7
239. Stephen-Haynes J, Gibson E. Principles of pressure ulcer management and prevention. Educational booklet 1 (4). Hartford, Huntingdon: *The Wound Care Society,* 2004.
240. National Institute for Clinical Excellence (NICE) (2001). Pressure ulcer risk assessment and prevention – Inherited Clinical Guideline B. ISBN: 1-84257083-8
241. National Institute for Clinical Excellence (NICE) (2001). Pressure ulcer risk assessment and prevention. A guide for patients and their carers. April
242. National Institute for Clinical Excellence (NICE) (2003). Pressure ulcer risk assessment and prevention and equipment selection
243. Pressure ulcer risk assessment and prevention. Implementation guide and protocol. Improving practice: improving care. RCN (2003), London
244. Wounds: Pressure ulcers. In Clinical Evidence. A compendium of the best available evidence for effective health care. BR MED J Publishing Group, issue 2, Dec 1999
245. Cooper JW. Psychoactive drugs may have a role in pressure sore origin. *BMJ* 2000; **321:** 452 (letter)
246. Landi F, Aloe L, Russo A *et al.* Topical treatment of pressure ulcers with nerve growth factor. *Ann Intern Med* 2003; **139:** 635–641
247. Langer G, Schloemer G, Knerr A, Kuss O, Behrens J. Nutritional interventions for preventing and treating pressure ulcers (Cochrane Review). In: The Cochrane Library, Issue 1, 2004. Chichester, UK: John Wiley & Sons, Ltd
248. Mustoe TA, Cooter RD, Gold MH, et al. International clinical recommendations on scar management. Plas. *Reconstr. Surg.* 2002; **110:** 560–571
249. Graham-Rowe D. Faster healing with fewer scars. *New Scientist* 2003: 21 June; 14
250. Jones JE, Nelson EA. Skin grafting for venous leg ulcers (Cochrane Review). In: The Cochrane Library, Issue 3, 2000. Oxford: Update Software

251. Bale S. A guide to wound debridement. *J Wound Care* 1997; **6:** 179–82
252. Tong A. The identification and treatment of slough. *J Wound Care* 1999; **8:** 338–9
253. Vowden KR, Vowden P. Wound debridement, Part 1: non-sharp techniques. *J Wound Care* 1999; **8:** 237–40
254. Vermeulen H, Ubbink D, Goossens A, de Vos R, Legemate D. Dressings and topical agents for surgical wounds healing by secondary intention. (Cochrane Review) In: The Cochrane Library, Issue 2, 2004, Chichester, UK: John Wiley & Sons, Ltd
255. Renton EJ. Pharmacological treatments for venous leg ulcers. *J Wound Care* 1999; **8**(4): 195–197
256. Briggs M, Nelson EA. Topical agents or dressings for pain in venous leg ulcers (Cochrane Review). In: Cochrane Library, Issue 3, 2000. Oxford: Update Software
257. De Araujo T, Valencia I, Federman DG, Kirsner RS. Managing the patient with venous ulcers. *Ann Intern Med.* 2003; **138:** 326–334
258. Barwell JR, Davies CE, Deacon J *et al.* Comparison of surgery and compression with compression alone in chronic venous ulceration (ESCHAR study): randomised controlled trial. *Lancet* 2004; **363:** 1854–59
259. The Canadian Coordinating Office for Health Technology Assessment. Pneumatic compression therapy on venous insufficiency. Jan 2004, No. 27 (www.ccohta.ca)
260. Morgan DA. Wound management products in the Drug Tariff. *Pharm J* 1999; **263:** 820–5
261. Morgan DA. The application of the 'ideal dressing' theory to practice. *Nursing Scotland* 1998; July: 16–18
262. National Prescribing Centre, Liverpool. Modern Wound Management Dressings. *Prescribing Nurse Bulletin* 1999; **1:** 5–8

VETERINARY SECTION

Small Animal Practice

by

Davina Anderson
MA VetMB PhD DSAS(ST) DipECVS MRCVS
European Specialist in Small Animal Surgery

Equine Practice

by

Emma Jones
MA VetMB CertES (Orth)

WOUND DRESSINGS IN SMALL ANIMAL PRACTICE

Wound healing in small animals

Wound healing in small animals (dogs and cats) is largely similar to the physiological processes seen in human patients.[1]

The vast majority of wounds seen in veterinary practice are as a result of traumatic injuries and the ischaemic distal limb injuries seen in human patients associated with diabetes mellitus or cardiovascular disease are extremely rare. In addition, dogs and cats do not develop clinical atherosclerosis, so the venous or arterial occlusive ischaemic diseases are also not seen. Otherwise the principles of wound management remain the same as in human wound management: necrotic or contaminated material must be removed, a clean moist environment must be maintained for granulation and epithelialisation. Contraction is an important part of the physiology of wound healing in dogs and cats due to the highly elastic and loose skin on the trunk. The slightly higher basal body temperature of dogs and cats mean that metabolic processes may occur faster and wound healing may progress quicker than in humans. The site specific issues of wound healing as seen in the horse do not occur in dogs and cats other than there being less loose skin available for contraction in the distal limb.

Functional repair of skin is the primary issue in veterinary wound management and scarring or cosmetic issues are of secondary importance to morbidity and distress caused by long term wound management. This is particularly important in nervous or aggressive patients where rapid final closure of wounds with a surgical procedure may be preferable to long term wound management.

Wound contraction is central to open wound management in dogs and cats. The skin on the trunk and neck is far more distensible and elastic than in human patients and contraction of wounds may contribute up to 30-50% to wound closure. So long as the contraction does not affect a body orifice or joint, this is seen as beneficial. The surrounding skin relaxes to allow for the increased tension and the movement of unaffected haired skin into the wounded area brings robust furred skin over the site which protects and conceals the scar. Occasionally severe contracture does cause functional problems particularly if burn wounds are allowed to heal by second intention, or the wound is fully circumferential on the distal limb.

Clinical management of veterinary patients

One of the big problems in veterinary wound management is that many patients are determined to remove their dressing – gnawing at the dressing, followed by damage and contamination of the wound is common. Urinary or faecal contamination of bandages also has to be prevented. There is the additional risk that the animal may consume the dressing and suffer a gastrointestinal obstruction, although this is rare.

Animals are often sedated or at least given analgesics prior to wound dressing and this means that daily dressings are difficult without long term hospitalisation. Owners put pressure on veterinary surgeons to allow discharge of the animal from the hospital, but home management of wound dressings is difficult because of the complexity of safe and effective bandaging of the lower limb in animals.[2] Animals may be managed as outpatients with regular visits for bandage changes, but in the early stages of wound management hospitalisation is ideal, allowing adequate analgesia and safe restraint for each dressing change.

Dressing requirements

Copious exudate is rarely seen in veterinary wounds, except in conditions of infection or presence of contaminated material or necrotic tissue. This means that high levels of fluid absorption by the dressing is less important than in human wound management. In fact, sometimes maintenance of a moist environment over granulation tissue may be more of an issue than fluid absorption. In addition, wound odour is not a significant problem unless severe wound infection occurs.

Dressings that are designed to adhere to the surrounding skin are difficult to apply in dogs and cats. These dressings adhere poorly to animals with large guard hairs such as Labrador Retrievers or Boxers. Animals with fine silky hairs such as Poodles or cats have a much smoother surface once the hair has been clipped, and the dressings adhere better.

There is no Drug Tariff system in veterinary medicine; veterinary surgeons and veterinary nurses are allowed to choose dressings and apply them as they see fit. Dressings that have been approved for use as medical devices in the human field are available for use in veterinary practice, without special licence. However those dressings that have been classified as pharmaceuticals can only be used at the clinical discretion of the veterinary surgeon under the 'cascade' system.[3] In real terms, most veterinary surgeons and nurses are only exposed to those dressings that the manufacturers have chosen to market in the veterinary field. The main player in this has been Smith and Nephew Healthcare who have the largest veterinary marketing section with specific veterinary literature, although the packaging is often the same or similar to that used for human patient use. There is currently no requirement in the UK for dressings only aimed at the veterinary market to be licensed, and the onus is on the manufacturer to ensure sterility and clinical efficacy. Sometimes a dressing is specifically labelled for veterinary use only.

Objective data on wound dressings in veterinary practice

The literature on dressings in small animal practice is sparse compared with the human field and there are no controlled prospective clinical trials for any dressing products. This is partly as a result of the costs involved compared with the revenue from the veterinary market and also due to the paucity of standardised wounds in clinical practice, as they are mostly traumatic. The controlled *in vivo* research largely comes from the Scott-Ritchey Research Centre at Auburn University in Alabama, USA.

Currently, Smith and Nephew Healthcare (Veterinary Division) supply the vast majority of the dressings on the veterinary market. However there are some products that are specifically available only to the veterinary profession (small animals) and these are listed below, with associated veterinary references and data, Many wound products that are regularly used by the veterinary profession, such as polyurethane foam dressings have no objective veterinary data available on their use.

Products marketed by Smith and Nephew Healthcare (Veterinary Division) for veterinary use include the following (**Table 1**), all of which are described in the main formulary.

Table 1. Products marketed for veterinary use.

Acticoat	Flamazine
Carbonet	Intrasite conformable
Exu-Dry	Intrasite Gel Applipak
Jelonet	Iodoflex
Melolin	Iodosorb
Primapore	Opsite Flexifix
Tricotex	Opsite Flexigrid
Aligisite-M	Opsite Incise
Allevyn trilaminate	Opsite IV3000
Allevyn bilaminate	Opsite Post-op
Allevyn Shaped	Opsite Spray
Allevyn Adhesive	Replicare ultra
Allevyn Cavity	Cica-care
Allevyn Hydrocellular	Skin prep
Cavi-care	Zoff

ACTIVATED CARBON DRESSINGS
Activate (RobinsonCare)
Although there is no evidence that odour is a problem with veterinary wounds, this product has been popular anecdotally for its wound management properties. A low adherent wound face with an activated charcoal cloth on the other side. The backing consists of a vapour permeable film and the outer layer is a non woven fabric. The dressing absorbs exudates and binds bacteria to the carbon fibres.

ALOE VERA (ACEMANNAN)[4, 5]
Anecdotal evidence of improved wound healing is abundant, but there are few controlled veterinary studies. The two studies cited found no significant difference in final healing rate of full thickness wounds, although wound strength at 21 days was higher in wounds treated with aloe vera. In one study, on the topical application of aloe vera, it was found that the early stages of wound healing in dog paw pad wounds were accelerated (first seven days) but that there was no overall difference.[4] Studies in research animals have shown that acemannan derived from aloe vera has enhanced wound healing.

Aloe vera veterinary formula, Aloe gelly (Forever Living Products)
Contains stabilised pure aloe vera gel. Aloe activator – an aloe vera and allantoin combination recommended for cleansing of wounds prior to application of aloe gelly. It has a pH of 4.5.

AMNION
Works as an occlusive dressing; equine amnion is normally used in preference to canine which is too thin.[6] The amnion contains antibacterial agents, lysozymes and allantoin, and full thickness wounds healed faster under amnion than under hydrogel or polyethylene. Amnion is cleaned by washing in dilute chlorhexidine prior to use and so long as the amnion is collected from a normal delivery (not a miscarriage which may be associated with infectious agents) there are no pathogens that can cross from the equine tissue to the dog or cat. It is not readily available.

COLLAGEN DRESSINGS
Collamend (Genitrix)
Available as particles, suspension (in a syringe ready for application) or a sheet dressing. Bovine Type I collagen. Designed to promote haemostasis, absorb wound fluid, contribute to wound strength and accelerate healing by providing an optimal environment for granulation tissue formation and epithelial migration. This product is licenced for veterinary use by the FDA in the USA as Medefil by BioCore Medical Technology Inc.

Vet-BIOSIST™ (Cooks)

Lyophilised porcine small intestinal submucosa dressing, not for use in humans. It is an acellular collagen-based material, consisting of Collagen types I, III and V, but is largely collagen type I. It also is a source of proteoglycans and glycosaminoglycans which serve as binding sites for growth factors. Early marketing aimed this at the wound management field but later marketing is now directed at its use as a biological material for reconstruction of hernias, body wall deficits, bladder and vessel augmentation. One study found no difference in the rate of healing over exposed bone than wounds dressed with polyethylene membrane.[7]

Emovet (BioLogic Nelson Veterinary Ltd)

A type 1 collagen dressing – promoted as a haemostatic agent and also a wound healing stimulant.

GARLIC

Garlic juice (Dorwest Herbs)

Veterinary product available for treatment of cuts and scratches and said to be safe on open wounds. However, there are no data on the use of garlic on wounds, although some of the products extracted from garlic may have antimycotic activity; pure garlic can cause skin burns.[8]

HYDROCOLLOIDS[9]

Granuflex (Convatec)

Evidence supporting use of hydrocolloid dressings in small animals is slim. Studies tend to find that the contraction is poor, healing rate may be slower and bacterial counts are higher. One study found that granulation tissue was 'grey' and atrophic or excessively exuberant slowing healing.[9] Another study suggested that contraction was inhibited under the hydrocolloid because adherence of the dressing to the wound edges 'splinted' the wound and prevented contraction from occurring which is generally a disadvantage in small animal wound healing.[10]

HYDROGELS

Aquaform (TSK Animal Health), Intrasite gel (S & N), Vetalintex (RobinsonCare)

Hydrogels are marketed in the veterinary field as a way to provide moist healing conditions while allowing for gentle debridement and absorption of exudates. The research evidence for management of (clean) full thickness wounds does not specifically indicate that it is much better than polyethylene dressings although it is much less adherent and this can be helpful in dressing changes in conscious animals. The anecdotal evidence from human patients concerning its analgesic properties may also help this. Personal communications – hydrogels have been used to soften fistulae with grass seeds in, to treat abscess cavities in rabbits and to reduce oedema in full thickness skin grafts.

NON/LOW ADHERENT DRESSINGS
Paraffin gauze dressings[10]
Grassolind (Millpledge), Jelonet (S & N)
These have been shown in a controlled study of healing of full thickness wounds in dogs to significantly delay epithelialisation, and the authors recommended the use of paraffin gauze only in early management of wounds. Grassolind is meant to be a stronger and more open lattice gauze base to improve performance and handling in veterinary use.

Polyethylene membrane[9, 6]
Skintact (RobinsonCare), Melolin (S & N), Rondopad (Millpledge)
Anecdotal evidence finds these dressings are often too dry for use in granulating wounds in dogs and cats. One study found little difference between the rate of healing of full thickness wounds in dogs under hydrogel or polyethylene dressings, although the hydrogel had a higher contraction epithelialisation ratio, and another found that wounds healed faster under the polyethylene dressing. These dressings are the standard dressing for use over surgical wounds that are bandaged and some practitioners trim them for use between the toes and under the first digit to protect normal skin from pressure excoriation and maceration when the limb is bandaged.

Rondopad (Millpledge)
A non/low adherent perforated film absorbent dressing. A thin absorbent layer of cellulosic and synthetic fibres backed with a strong non-woven material cover, then bonded to a polyester film on both surfaces which is evenly perforated.

LP dressing pads (Millpledge)
A leak-proof pad of a sleeve of soft non-woven light material covering a padded filling of 100% absorbent cotton wool with a moisture repellent barrier film inside the back surface of the pad. The edges are all sealed so the cotton wool cannot come out during use.

Sanipore-strip (Millpledge)
Central low-adherent dressing pad backed with a conforming stretch adhesive backing.

SILVER DRESSINGS OR COATED DRESSINGS[11]
Acticoat (S & N), Flamazine (S & N)
An equine *in vitro* study showed that silver dressings had a significant antibacterial effect. The effect was time dependent and not concentration dependent. Long-lasting antibacterial effects *in vivo* that do not cause increased risk of multi-drug resistant bacteria may be useful in cases where infection would be devastating (e.g. decubital ulcers in the presence of orthopaedic implants) and may help reduce the use of long term antibiotic therapy in veterinary practice.

SPRAY DRESSINGS
Op-site Spray (S & N)
Dermaflex spray dressing (Lohmann)
Antiseptic spray wound dressing forms a protective layer protecting the wound from flies and dirt. Used on sutured surgical wounds that cannot be dressed as well as superficial open wounds.

Cavilon™ (3M)
Hexamethyldisiloxane and polyethenylmethylsiloxane acrylate co-polymer spray. Forms a transparent waterproof protective film on the skin. Alcohol free and non-sting, even when applied to inflamed skin. It stretches with skin movement and remains intact for 48-72 hours. It is recommended to protect skin under adhesive tapes or to protect skin from urine and faecal contact. Anecdotally has also been an effective treatment for acute moist dermatitis (common in dogs).

Film dressing spray (Millpledge)
A transparent spray used to seal surgical wounds.

SUGARS AND HONEY
There is a small amount of information available for their use in veterinary medicine, two recent review articles are referenced.[12, 13]

TRIPEPTIDE-COPPER COMPLEX
Glycyl-L-histidyl—L-lysine tripeptide-copper complex has been shown to accelerate healing in canine chronic wounds in rats possibly via inhibition of TNF-alpha.[14] However in another study, TCC showed no significant difference to saline in paw pad wounds, although they healed better in the later stages than those treated with acemannan (aloe vera derived immunostimulant).[5]

Tris-EDTA[15]
Has been used to cleanse infected wounds and to potentiate the effects of antibiotics and antiseptics, particularly on resistant bacteria. It has been used in the treatment of chronic fistula and aural lavage in the dog. (1.2g EDTA, 6.05g tris in 1 litre of sterile water, pH adjusted to 8.0 with dilute NaOH. This solution is then autoclaved).

POULTICES AND COMPRESSES
Animalintex (RobinsonCare)
The only product available specifically for poulticing. It consists of Tragocanth (poulticing agent) and Boric acid (an antiseptic), and is recommended for use in horses or dogs for hot or cold poulticing. It may cause maceration of intact skin and should be used with care in small animals.

Vet-ice wraps (Millpledge)
Lightweight sheet or wrap made up of two layers of a tough unique one-way permeable material sandwiched together and evenly cross-bonded at intervals to create rows of compartments, each 5cm, square. Each cell contains an inert dry powder which has the ability to absorb up to ten times its weight of water or aqueous fluids, swelling to create a soft pliable gel. The gel is non-toxic and inert and cannot leak from the cells. The sheets or sachets may then be heated or cooled for a variety or hot or cold pack uses. It is flexible and conforming, holds the temperature for a long time and can be re-used.

ADDRESSES

3M Healthcare Ltd, 3M House, Morley Street, Loughborough, Leics LE11 1EP

Arnolds Veterinary Products Ltd., Cartmel Drive, Harlescott, Shrewsbury, Shropshire, SY1 3TB (Distributor)

Cooks Veterinary Products (UK) Ltd., Monroe House, GB-Letchworth, Herts, SGG 1LN

Dorwest Herbs, Shipton Gorge, Bridport, Dorset, DT6 4LP

Forever Living Products, The Oaks, Manor Farm Court, Swaffham Prior, Cambridge, CB5 0JL.

Genitrix Ltd., Forest Road, Horsham, West Sussex, RH12 4HL

Millpledge, Whinley Estate, Clarborough, Retford, Notts, DN22 9NA

Nelson Veterinary Ltd., Manor Farm, Winstone, Cirencester, Glos, GL7 7JU

Robinson, Lawn Road, Carlton-in-Lindrick, Industrial Estate, Worksop, Nottinghamshire, S81 9LB

TSK Animal Health Ltd., Mill Close, Brompton, Bedale, North Yorkshire, DL8 1JY.

REFERENCES

1. Dyson M. Advances in wound healing physiology: the comparative perspective. *Vet Derm* 1997; **8:** 227–233.
2. Anderson DM, White RAS. Ischaemic bandage injuries: a retrospective study in nine dogs and two cats. A review and discussion of the literature. *Vet Surg* 2000; **29:** 488–498.
3. The use of veterinary medicinal products. In: Guide to Professional Conduct: Hawksmere; 2002. p. 39.
4. Swaim SF, Riddell KP, McGuire JA. Effects of topical medications on the healing of open pad wounds in dogs. *JAAHA* 1992; **28:** 499–502.
5. Swaim SF, Vaughn DM, Kincaid SA, Morrison NE, Murray SS, Woodhead MA, *et al*. Effects of locally injected medications on healing pad wounds in dogs. *JAVMA* 1996; **57:** 394–399.
6. Ramsey DT, Pope ER, Wagner-Mann C, Berg JN, Swaim SF. Effects of three occlusive dressing materials on healing of full-thickness skin wounds in dogs. *Am J Vet Res* 1995; **56**(7): 941–949.
7. Winkler JT, Swaim SF, Sartin EA, Henderson RA, Welch JA. The effect of a porcine-derived small intestinal submucosa product on wounds with exposed bone in dogs. *Vet Surg* 2002; **31**(6): 541–551.
8. Baruchin AM, Sagi A, Yoffe B, Ronen M. Garlic Burns. *Burns* 2001; **27**(7): 781–782.
9. Morgan PW, Binnington AG, Miller CW, Smith DA, Valliant A, Prescott JF. The effect of occlusive and semi-occlusive dressings on the healing of acute full thickness skin wounds on the forelimbs of dogs. *Vet Surg* 1994; **23:** 494–502.
10. Lee AH, Swaim SF, Yang ST, Wilken LO, Miller DP, Wilt GR, *et al*. The effects of petrolatum, polyethylene glycol, nitrofurazone, and a hydroactive dressing on open wound healing. *JAAHA* 1986; **22:** 443–451.
11. Adams AP, Santschi EM, Mellancamp MA. Antibacterial properties of a silver chloride-coated nylon wound dressing. *Vet Surg* 1999; **28:** 219–225.
12. Mathews KA, Binnington AG. Wound Management using honey. *Comp Cont Ed Vet* 2002; **24**(1): 53–60.
13. Mathews KA, Binnington AG. Wound Management using sugar. *Comp Cont Ed Vet* 2002; **24**(1): 41–50.
14. Canapp SO, Farese JP, Schultz GS, Swaim SF, VanGilder JM, Lee-Ambrose L, *et al*. The effect of topical tripeptide-copper complex in a model for chronic open wounds. In: Twelfth Annual American College of Veterinary Surgeons Symposium; 2002; San Diego: *Veterinary Surgery*; 2002. p. 478.
15. Ashworth CD, Nelson DR. Antimicrobial potentiation of irrigation solutions containing tris-[hydroxymethyl] aminomethane-EDTA. *JAVMA* 1990; **197**(11): 1513–1514.

WOUND DRESSINGS IN EQUINE PRACTICE

Wound healing in horses

Wound management is an important part of equine practice. Correct management can significantly reduce the time taken for wounds to heal and improve the welfare of our patients.

Traumatic injuries, particularly of the distal limb, are common in horses. External trauma (e.g. a kick by a field companion) is a frequent occurrence; abrasions (e.g. falling on a tarmac surface) are also common. Equine clinicians rarely see the dramatic degloving injuries seen by our small animal colleagues as road traffic accidents involving horses are thankfully infrequent.

Despite differences in aetiology, the basic physiological mechanisms of wound repair are similar between species. Management of this process is aimed at controlling the inflammatory phase using lavage to reduce contamination and careful debridement of devitalised tissue, then providing an optimal environment for granulation, epithelialisation, contraction and maturation to proceed.

Wound contraction is an important factor in equine wound healing. The skin of the neck and trunk is capable of a considerable degree of contraction with up to 70% of the skin deficit eliminated by this mechanism. Healing by wound contraction results in excellent cosmetic and functional repair. The functional limitations seen in human patients due to excessive wound contraction are generally not seen in horses, probably due to the amount of loose skin available and the expansibility of the surrounding skin. Significantly, wounds of the distal limb of horses demonstrate less contraction than wounds to the body. Recent studies have also shown that the skin on the distal limb of horses has a smaller capacity for contraction when compared with ponies, due to differences in the magnitude of the initial inflammatory response. This makes wound management in the distal limb of horses a particular challenge.

The clinical management of equine patients.

Aims of treatment

Many of our equine patients are required to perform as athletes and a return to function is of paramount importance. Some horses may also be used as show animals and therefore the cosmetic outcome is of importance to the owner. The owner's expectations should be clearly assessed early in the process of wound management. Procedures such as skin grafting should be considered if an excellent cosmetic result is required.

Practical factors

Patient restraint is a consideration common to both large and small animal wound management. In horses, repetitive general anaesthesia is problematic; not only is there a risk associated with anaesthesia, but a difficult recovery may result in further damage to the wound site. In the vast majority of horses, wound management and bandage changes can be achieved using standing chemical restraint.

Cost is also a major issue in the management of equine wounds. Due to the size of the animal and the labour intensive nature of wound management, the cost of treatment, even in uncomplicated cases, can rise rapidly.

As many of our patients will injure themselves while 'turned out', there may be a delay in detection of the injury and wound contamination may be significant. Therefore, despite the ideal situation of early return to function, wound management by second intention healing is necessary in the management of these wounds. Careful wound debridement and lavage is required. Large volume lavage with sterile isotonic saline at a pressure of 10–20psi will remove contaminants without forcing bacteria deeper into tissues. The importance of careful wound preparation at this stage cannot be over-estimated as it is believed that factors that prolong the inflammatory phase of wound healing predispose to the formation of exuberant granulation tissue.

Exuberant granulation tissue.

The over production of granulation tissue, occasionally seen in other species, is a common problem in distal limb wounds in horses. Excess granulation tissue is formed so that the outline of the tissue defect becomes convex, commonly referred to as 'proud flesh'. Once exuberant granulation tissue has formed, the process of epithelialisation is severely slowed and the excess tissue must be removed to allow wound healing to continue. This is best achieved by sharp resection. Although the application of caustic topical agents is common, it is difficult to ensure these chemicals do not contact the delicate epithelial cells and retard the healing process further. Corticosteroid creams are commonly applied to prevent the granulation tissue reforming; however again these agents will dramatically slow epithelialisation if they contact the wound edges.

Little research has been done into which wound dressings reduce the incidence of exuberant granulation tissue formation. However, it is generally accepted that minimal movement of the injured region will reduce the rate of granulation tissue formation. Therefore, correct bandage application is crucial in the management of distal limb wounds in horses.

The recent development of lightweight durable casting materials has significantly improved our ability to immobilise and support the equine distal limb. Cast application has become a practical and successful asset in the management of severe distal limb wounds.

FURTHER READING

Bertone AL, Sullins KE, Stashak TS, and Norrdin RW. Effect of wound location and the use of topical collagen gel on exuberant granulation tissue formation and wound healing in the horse and pony. *Am J Vet Res* 1985; **46**(7):1438–1444.

Wilmink JM, Stolk PW, Weeren PR and Barneveld A. Differences in second-intention wound healing between horses and ponies: macroscopical aspects. *Equine Vet* 1999; **J 31:** 53–60.

Wilmink JM, Weeren PR, Stolk PW, Van Mil FN and Barneveld A. Differences in second-intention wound healing between horses and ponies:histiological aspects. *Equine Vet* 1999; **J 31:** 61–67.

Wilmink JM, Henderbragt H, Weeren PR, Stolk PW, and Barneveld A. Differences in wound contraction between horses and ponies: the in vitro contraction capacity of fibroblasts. *Equine Vet J* 2001; **33:** 499–505.